GROUPWORK
ACTIVITIES

Dedication
To my parents

GROUPWORK ACTIVITIES

The resource
manual for everyone
working with elderly people

◆

Danny Walsh

First published in 1993 by
Winslow Press Ltd, Telford Road, Bicester, Oxon OX6 0TS, UK
www.winslow-press.co.uk
Reprinted 1994, 1995, 1996, 1997, 1998, 1999

Typeset by Gecko Limited, Bicester, Oxon

002-1724/Printed in Great Britain/1010

British Library Cataloguing in Publication Data
Walsh, Danny
    Groupwork Activities: The Resource Manual or Everyone Working
    With Elderly People
    I. Title
    6.18.97

ISBN 0 86388 120 3

Contents

About the Author

Danny Walsh was born in Lincolnshire and trained as a psychiatric nurse in Yorkshire. An interest in elderly care and groupwork arose as a response to the paucity of resources for this client group and also due to the wisdom and humanity that such groups have shared with him. He is currently the manager of a day hospital for elderly people suffering from psychiatric problems. He is married and has one son.

Acknowledgements

I would have liked to put these at the end of the book as it is only when you finish something that you realise you could not possibly have done it on your own. Many of the ideas here have been road tested at the Silkstream Day Hospital, Colindale. My thanks are due to the imagination and enthusiasm of the staff there — Mimi, Meg, Marina, Jackie, Elaine, Alice, Virginia, Anne and Shirin; this book is as much a result of their efforts as of mine. I am also grateful for the support of Keith Mellors who, as my manager, allowed the staff and myself the autonomy to develop unhindered but gave us much encouragement throughout.

Lesley Wilson, our consultant, has been a vital source of support. Her enthusiasm and wisdom have made the difference between being supported and feeling supported. Thank you.

I must also acknowledge Heather Gray who, having had to decipher my hieroglyphics, then type, retype and type again, still had to bear the burden of being my wife. Finally, my son Jake, for rearranging most of the chapters; by tearing up several and eating many pages I hope that he has proved the book to be largely digestible.

Danny Walsh

Foreword

Society is always changing and ours is no different, especially with respect to the proportion of the population that is old. Danny Walsh's book is therefore timely and relevant.

Increasing numbers of older people, many of them with significant mental health problems, will find themselves in day or residential care, and as Danny points out one day this will include us. If this experience is in any sense to be enjoyable or of benefit to older people then they will need the opportunity of exposure to a wide range of activities that can be tailored to their particular strengths, as well as their disabilities.

This book will be an invaluable resource to workers in the independent sector of care provision, as well as those within health and social services settings who wish to enhance the quality of the care they offer. It is a privilege for me to be asked to introduce it to you.

Dr Lesley Wilson
Consultant in Old Age Psychiatry
Silk Stream Unit, Colindale Hospital, London

Preface

This book contains a huge collection of tried and tested groupwork ideas covering a wide range of subjects. The reason for doing this is simply that I got sick of having to draw on ideas from hundreds of different sources . . . "if only they were all in one book!"

However this is not a manual on how to do groupwork. There are plenty of good books on the theory and practice of groupwork. Concerning elderly people I would point group leaders towards *Groupwork with the Elderly* (Bender et al, 1987), a very useful, but what's more, a very practical book. None the less I feel it is important that I should include a brief discussion of some of the virtues and pitfalls common to groupwork and these are to be found in Sections B and I of this book.

During testing I found that EMI (elderly mentally ill and infirm) groups derived great benefit from these activities and I have therefore included detailed advice on working with this often-neglected group.

Above all the emphasis is on fun. If there is one predisposing factor which makes a good groupworker it is a sense of humour and no amount of groupwork training can compensate for a lack of it.

Section A

SETTING THE SCENE

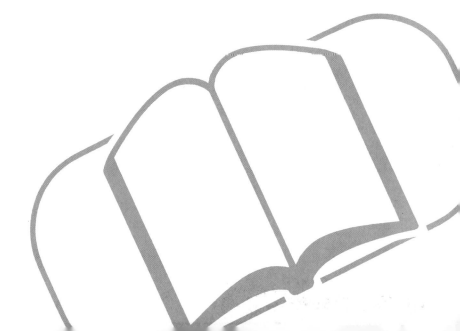

This book is intended as a practical guide, a resource for various groupwork activities which are of value when working with elderly people. The activities are suitable for any group of elderly people, but I have found them particularly rewarding when used in the sphere of old age psychiatry.

For far too long elderly mentally ill and infirm people have been victims of a lack of resources, regarded as low priority, deemed beyond meaningful interaction and unreceptive to stimulation. It is high time this group of people were given the time, skilled intervention and quality of life they deserve. One aim of this manual is to foster this goal and therefore there are copious notes and hints on how to work with such specialized groups.

WHY BOTHER?

Question: Why bother about groupwork with elderly mentally ill people?

Answer: The proportion of elderly people in society is rising; consequently so is the number suffering from dementia and other mental illnesses.

Most dementing elderly people are, and will continue to be, cared for at home. Presently only about 20 per cent of sufferers are cared for in hospitals or other institutions. The relatives want to look after their loved ones at home, but they need support. The great majority of these carers are the spouses of the sufferers and pensioners themselves. There is therefore a great immediate need for more day care provision. Whilst providing respite for carers, it should also provide meaningful and stimulating activity for the sufferers. It is within this setting as well as in institutions that good

groupwork becomes profoundly important.

It is easier to let go and let others look after your loved one if you know that they will be receiving the loving care that you expect for them and know that they will be stimulated during that time by mixing with others in meaningful group activity.

If we look also at elderly people suffering from functional psychiatric illnesses such as depression we can see again a major role for groupwork which focuses on social and inter-action skills. For elderly people in general relationships often deteriorate and social skills are lost due to isolation and loneliness. They don't get the chance to practise those skills. If the situation is compounded by psychiatric illness we also have additional factors of:

- ◆ withdrawal
- ◆ shunning by others due to bizarre behaviour
- ◆ paranoia (suspicion of others)
- ◆ anxiety
- ◆ fear of failure
- ◆ effects of institutionalization
- ◆ depression
- ◆ feelings of worthlessness
- ◆ loss of self-esteem
- ◆ loss of confidence
- ◆ stigma from others

Even where we have bothered about elderly mentally ill people we haven't bothered much about groupwork. We give a service of sorts but the quality is often sadly lacking.

A report in 1980 called *Time for Action* (Godlove & Rodwell) highlighted the deficits here. It showed that day centres and day hospitals provide much more contact with others than do hospital wards and residential homes. Groupwork is a prime factor in increasing this contact time.

In this research, however, most of the 'time spent with others' was merely 'sitting' or other 'informal recreation' — only a small percentage (23.5 per cent in day centres and 11.3 per cent in day hospitals) was spent in organized activity. However, contact with others — either physical or verbal —during these activities was minimal: 4.7 per cent of the time in day centres and 2.7 per cent in day hospitals.

So here again is another reason for bothering with groupwork in our chosen context.

Our purpose is to provide a list and explanations of a wide range of groupwork activities in order to show that there is more to life than knitting woolly poodles and watering the geraniums. Many of the activities will increase that all important 'contact time with others' and, it is hoped, they are all good fun as well. Having fun and being old have a lot in common, they are both under-rated and given far too low a priority.

Mental illness in old age is not a barrier to groupwork; it does not render the sufferer incapable of being stimulated and does not severely limit the possibilities for effective groupwork.

The skill, in any form of groupwork, lies in pitching it at the right level.

We all lie at different points on the continuum between being mentally healthy and mentally unwell and we move back and forth along this line throughout our lives. One day the dog dies, the next day you win the pools.

Likewise we are also variable in our receptiveness to groupwork. If I suffer from dementia it means you need to adapt your approach to me because clearly some of my abilities, notably short-term memory, orientation and communication skills are affected. If I have had a particularly bad dose of the blues, and been deemed clinically depressed, then none of my intellectual faculties have been altered permanently, but you will need to understand how I feel and tailor the group to suit my needs accordingly.

It may well be that the group is the most important part of my treatment if I am ever to crawl out of this hole I find myself in.

The target for this book then is anyone working with elderly people with mental health problems, whether the difficulties stem from dementia, psychosis or neurosis. It is aimed at hospital nurses, community nurses, residential social workers, social workers, care assistants, voluntary workers, relatives and carers.

I am writing this from the point of view of a day hospital for elderly people suffering problems of mental health, but this does not prevent the application of the principles to groups organized elsewhere.

What then can groupwork do? In general it reduces the sense of isolation that many feel. Participating in regular group activity fosters a sense of belonging and togetherness.

It can also:

◆ give peer support

◆ be an information exchange

◆ be an opportunity to take an in-depth look at ourselves and compare this to how others see us

◆ combat demoralization with mutual support

◆ increase self-esteem

◆ give us a role

◆ increase self-knowledge

◆ confront dubious or mistaken ideas of reality

◆ give the opportunity to learn to trust others

◆ help us recognize that our problems are not unique

◆ help us discover alternative strategies

◆ increase our independence

◆ give us the opportunity to share problems

◆ give us the opportunity to learn new and rekindle old social skills

◆ provide us with a safe arena in which to practise social skills

◆ give us a sense of achievement

◆ allow us to take risks in an uncritical atmosphere

◆ allow us to practise self-expression safely

◆ allow us to make mistakes without the fear of looking and feeling stupid

◆ be fun

A friend once told me, and I'm inclined to agree, that everyone should be in a group. Indeed most of us are in several groups: family, work, peers and so on; but all of us could gain valuable personal insights from belonging to a 'therapeutic', 'awareness', 'growth' (call it what you will) type of group.

GROUPS FOR DEMENTING ADULTS

Whilst short-term memory may be lost and skills such as putting clothes on in the right order may have gone, many dementia sufferers retain skills which have been learnt in earlier years and practised over a long period of time, such as playing the piano, the words of old songs, a sense of rhythm and dancing. Also social skills, attitudes and qualities such as good naturedness and manners often remain intact until the final stages of the illness.

Recognizing and focusing on these skills is very important: it is a recognition of individuality and self-worth.

A few examples:
One client who attends our day hospital regularly will not key into much of what we do: "This is bloody silly, it's childish," she will say while we are looking at slides and talking about holidays and places we have been. She usually walks out, and this is her right. That is the reality for her and she is above it. Word games using a blackboard meet with the same response: "Bloody childish, we're not school kids." But, bring out the old sing-along-a-Max and hey

presto — "you are my sunshine" — she loves it, she remembers all the words, sings away merrily, and is very capable of being winked at, flattered and asked for the next dance. She becomes blissfully happy and quite a flirt — "You saucy bugger," she will say, giving me a crafty wink. The important point here is you have found something — music, song and dance — that makes this lady very happy, recognizes her considerable skill and fosters it. So we learn we can include her in other sessions — just bring out the Max Bygraves tapes and she will enjoy herself whilst you carry on with the group, giving her regular feedback, singing along with her now and again or just winking at each other. Groupwork skill no. 17 — winking!

Another gets much out of any group if you can involve her social skills. She becomes a hostess — which is what she is good at and what she wants to be. She will join in any activity but all she wants is the opportunity to be gracious.

Conversely another client may need peace and quiet and not function in a group setting at all: it can be confusing, noisy and frightening.

You must know your clients as individuals and act upon that knowledge accordingly.

It is crucial to take into account their levels of ability before you merrily indulge in any activity. The activity should be geared to their level of competence so that it is:

1 not so easy as to induce feelings of ridicule, childishness and patronization, or

2 so hard as to induce feelings of failure and frustration.

INSIGHT

One of the most devastating phases of dementia is that period in which, for many, they have some degree of insight into their disintegrating mind.

They know they are forgetful, and know they do apparently 'silly things'. They must feel inadequate, silly, a burden, stupid, hopeless, scared stiff about what is happening to them, and horrified and embarrassed as to what other people might think of them. For these people I plead a special case. Here it may be better to have arrived than to still be travelling. The person who is profoundly demented, or at least beyond insight, probably has none of the above psychological traumas; although we cannot be certain of this. Fear and frustration may still be evident. However, it remains true that for those who possess insight there should be separate groups.

Never 'lump' them together with those whose dementia is beyond insight. The level of skill in the group, for one thing, will be far too wide and those with insight will merely receive terrible reminders of what they are probably about to become and will think that you feel they are that deteriorated already. It can only cause them grief and much deep sadness.

Section B

INTERACTION & SELF-EXPLORATION

An important part of groupwork is the period before the group starts. In a day hospital or centre, for half an hour to an hour after clients arrive there is a period of welcoming, relaxing, having a cup of tea and setting the tone and atmosphere. The clients are greeted and greet each other: "Hello, great to see you, how are you, what have you been up to this week?" Each is made to feel relaxed and at ease with the staff and with each other. This fosters feelings of belonging, being wanted, self-esteem, self-worth, and is an unstructured, very loose social skills exercise. Most importantly, though, it sets the tone for the day — relaxed and non-threatening. In residential and in-patient settings, the same applies. Starting the group with a relaxed cup of tea after the busy morning schedule of rising and breakfasting, again, sets the tone. Ask "Did you have a good night's sleep?" or "Did you enjoy the music last night?"

Similarly, after lunch, the siesta performs the same function. Lunch is for many elderly people a highlight of the day to be savoured at leisure and staff should sit down and share this experience. I know of one 'place' where the person in charge even goes through the menu — 'colour co-ordinating' it — adding a few carrots or peas to perk up an otherwise dismal monotone plate. Her worst nightmare was a plate of fish in white sauce with cauliflower and mashed potatoes. She has a point, the meal is an occasion — use it.

The end of the day, winding down, preparing to go, is also an important period. It is an opportunity again to practise social skills, bid farewells, and care must be taken to end the day in a relaxed and happy manner. People should want to come back next week, not feel that they have to.

Again in 'long stay' settings this is equally important, if not more so. Focus on the day's achievements: "That's the third time in a row you've beaten me at chess, Tom." Groups in residential settings are crucial if one day is not to blur into the next. Our own lives may be routine but they are varied by the idiosyncrasies of work, family life and mobility. The question we must ask is how we can make tomorrow different from today for Tom.

This is really for a group which meets regularly and whose composition does not change very often.

This group takes place in the morning, it is the first group of the day and serves several purposes.

It brings the whole community together which is, in itself, important, as opposed to sitting in isolated groups or individually about the place. Merely sitting in as part of the meeting will give those who tend to isolate themselves a sense of belonging. That their presence is required underlines the fact that they are a valued member of the group. Those who walk out or will not attend should not be ignored. Group members should go out and ask them to join, emphasizing that they are being missed and that their presence and contributions are wanted by the rest of the group. It is important, however, to recognize and respect an individual's autonomy. There are many valid reasons for not wanting interaction or the company of others and this should never be forced upon anybody. Privacy and isolation are a right and a privilege that most of us hold dear. For the majority of us these are relatively easy to achieve, but in a residential, or a long-stay setting, such targets may be desperately difficult to achieve. A single room is all too often a luxury, and going to the toilet might be the only time you are truly alone, but if there are thirty other residents even this luxury may be short-lived!

Back with the group, however; it exists for its members to say 'hello' to each other every day and to set the day's agenda, discussing what will happen later in the day.

Once the group is settled, it should concentrate on building cohesiveness by focusing on current (here and now) feelings. For example: "Bill is leaving tomorrow, I'm going to miss him"; or "I'm really glad that Henry is joining in more."

Feelings can be explored which are common to group members. Mutual support is gained when we see others in similar situations to ours and hear how they feel and cope. Much isolation can be reduced in this way.

The group welcomes new members and discusses fears and thoughts regarding coming into hospital, residential care or attending the group for the first time.

The many fears and problems arising from impending discharge from hospital can be highlighted.

The group leader strives to encourage members to concentrate on the feelings that are being experienced during the group. It is important that outside issues are not allowed to take over the group and that it does not decline into a 'has the kettle been mended yet?' type of meeting. The leader must point out that these issues can and should be raised outside the group.

The sense of community and belonging that this group fosters lays the foundations for more directly therapeutic interventions.

The group is useful as well in the once a week setting of a day hospital or other situation. When a regular group has developed, sharing the issues of your week is very supportive and it can be the most directly therapeutic group of the day. It is up to the group leader to decide how therapeutic the group should be and how deep it should go; only they have the knowledge of what stage the group is at, how cohesive it is and what it can 'take'.

It is possible in this setting to gradually build a more directly therapeutic group which tackles key problem areas, from one which begins fairly innocuously. It ought to be said, though, that if this is your intention it should be made clear to the participants in advance of their joining the group.

I deliberately have not included many warm-ups because most of the interaction activities which follow can be adapted for use as warm-ups, so we are left with three which can withstand constant repetition.

WHAT THE PAPERS SAY

There are many things which can be gleaned from a newspaper as a way of getting the brain kickstarted in the morning. For a group which includes those whose sight is not too good, a newspaper which has large headlines and good, preferably colour, photos is useful.

Examples:

1 Whose birthday it is

2 Read a country diary to remind us of nature's seasonal activities

3 Focus on and discuss or just admire particularly good photographs

4 The major headlines of course can be discussed

5 Any local issues

6 What the royals are up to

7 What everyone else is up to, and who with (tabloids)

8 Sporting news

9 Politics

10 Horoscopes

11 Weather forecast

12 Twenty-five and fifty years ago — many papers run small sections detailing news stories of yesteryear.

There are of course many more things you can glean and later we will delve deeper with regard to discussion groups.

ON THIS DAY IN HISTORY

This is a very useful book by Simon Mayo that we use all the time as a quick warm-up, but it can also be used as a group exercise in its own right.

Basically for each day of the year it highlights birthdays, deaths and famous events that have occurred on that day in history.

It reminds us of the day, and it is interesting to locate what events happened and whose birthday it is. Don't get too carried away with its reality orientation possibilities, though — it is all very well saying that today is Sunday August 26th 1993, but when you start chatting about how Julius Caesar invaded Britain in 55BC and the island of Krakatoa began to erupt in 1883 and Queen Victoria's husband Prince Albert was born in 1819 and so on, it can get a bit confusing . . . Prince Albert is 174 years old today!

CUSHION THROW

This is good for getting to know people's names, checking on memories and is useful exercise.

Sit in a tight circle and pass the cushion around to the right, saying the name of the person to whom you are giving it, then go to the left doing the same. Next throw the cushion to anybody in the circle, saying the name of the person to whom you are throwing it. Try and get the cushion flying around all over the place and keep it up for a minute or two.

If you are feeling really enthusiastic and everyone else is enjoying it, start throwing a second cushion around as well.

ACTIVITIES

The emphasis here, while there is often an underlying therapeutic value, is on bringing people together. Interaction groups serve the purpose of giving meaningful activity, which is enjoyable and helps bring about group cohesiveness, thereby laying the foundations for more therapeutic group activities. They help to enhance a feeling of togetherness and promote a sense of community in hospital wards and other institutional settings. They can be adapted for a particular clientele and for the particular stage a group has reached. They are also valuable in drawing in the more isolated and withdrawn members of the group, the facilitator being able to vary the depth of a game from a fairly superficial, non-threatening exercise to a more personal form of interaction involving greater degrees of self-expression and self-exposure.

Most interaction groups also function as a focus and practice ground for social skills. It is important that the facilitator understands exactly what their goals are for the group and just what it is they wish to achieve. This being so, it is equally important that the activities lie within the skill range of the group and thus the objectives are achievable in order for members to attain a degree of success and pride in that success. More therapeutic interactions involving personal disclosure should not be introduced early on in a group's life, but later when the group has achieved a sufficient degree of trust in order for members to explore feelings in a safe environment. Fun is again to the fore among desirable objectives and need not detract in any way from the more therapeutic objectives.

Many of the group activities described in later sections can be used as the basis for interaction groups, most notably those from the section on 'perception games'. It is for the facilitator to decide what to use and when to use it.

KNOTS

This was one of the first group exercises I was ever introduced to and the one that got me hooked. It is great fun but needs fairly fit and active clients.

Ask members to stand in a circle shoulder to shoulder and squeeze up tight together. Then tell them to close their eyes and reach out with both hands to the centre of the circle. Ask them to get hold of two other hands and when everyone has got hold of two other sweaty palms tell them to open their eyes. You might need to adjust one or two hands, or help stray hands find partners so that you don't have clusters of three or four hands together. What you have now is a human knot with arms interwoven. Inform the group that it is nearly always possible to untangle this knot without anyone letting go of any one else's hand.

Tell them to get on with it, sit back and giggle away quietly to yourself as you enjoy the ensuing chaos. Members will be pleasantly surprised when they eventually find it can be done.

IF THEY WERE A FLOWER

For me this is the standard by which I measure all other interaction games, not just with elderly people but any group. It is not always possible to do with some groups as it demands a certain degree of abstract thought but it is by no means unachievable and can be adapted to do away with the abstract. It is very useful, given a good facilitator, with groups of clients overcoming the debilitating effects of depression, which so often leaves our self-esteem in tatters. As a group it is enjoyable and provides a useful insight into how we see ourselves and how others see us. It is based loosely on Johari's window, of which more later (see page 34).

After you have warmed up and the group is settled ask one member of the group to be 'it'. Ask 'it' to think of another member of the group but not to tell us. When ready the rest of the group is invited to put one question to 'it' such as:

"If the person were a flower what flower would it be?"

Each has a turn using categories like car, cake, animal, plant, noise, colour, texture, piece of clothing and so on.

This goes on until someone thinks they know who it is. They say who and why they think it is that person. "Oh, so you think I'm a pink poodle do you? Thanks a million."

Usually we give each other positive feedback, saying relatively good things and it is nice to have complimentary things said about you, especially when you are depressed and think you are pretty worthless.

These positive comments are what one psychologist I met once called 'warm fluffies'. We need 'warm fluffies', she would say, because we are only getting 'cold nasties' most of the time. Back in our game we seldom get comments of the 'cold nasty' kind, like "I guessed it was you . . . colour — grey, animal — slug . . . because you're slow and slimy." Thank goodness; but we can and do get feedback about the way others see us and it is very interesting to see this side of ourselves. "I didn't realize people felt that about me", "I never thought I came across like that", "Is that how you think I am?"

So we have got a very enjoyable and also a very stimulating and disclosing game. As the group leader you must retain control and make the game as superficial or deep as is appropriate.

UNDER A FIVER

The object here is to sell yourself. Place an advert in the local paper's 'under a fiver' column in order to try and sell yourself; for example, 'vegetarian male, one previous owner, bodywork shabby but low mileage, runs on Guinness, loves the countryside.'

Get everyone to write one of these; do not take too long about it. Then ask them to fold the paper several times and throw it into the bin which you have thoughtfully provided in the middle of the group (groupwork skill no. 127 — make sure the bin is empty).

Shake the bin (no real need for this but the exercise will do you good) and pass it around, asking everyone to take a piece of paper out. Then go around and say who you think it is and why . . . maybe even make them an offer.

FACE GUESS

A bit more active this one and one that could also come under 'perception games'. It is good, though, as an interaction to break the ice and get things livened up a bit.

Ask someone to be 'it'. Sit them on a chair in the middle of the group and blindfold them. Take them by the hand and lead them around the chair a few times to disorient them so that they cannot remember who is sitting where. Then lead them up to another member of the group and place their hands on that person's face. They must simply guess whose face they are touching . . . great fun!

HUMAN NOUGHTS AND CROSSES

This involves two teams and nine chairs in a square, three by three, close together. Then just play noughts and crosses with team members linking hands when placed in position. Again this is a good one to use either as a warm-up, to liven things up or as a relaxer, after a 'thinking' game.

NAMES

With the group sat in a close circle, go round saying what your name is, any middle names, why you were called that, and what you think about it. Do you like it or loathe it? Have you any nicknames? What would you like to have been called? You can look up the names in a book; they are usually marked as books of 'babies' names', but they tell you what the name means and where it is derived from.

BIRTHDAYS

This is another interesting session based on Simon Mayo's book, *On this Day in History*.

Just go around asking each member when their birthday is and read out what famous events have their anniversaries on that day and with whom they share their birthdays. People are usually quite surprised to learn these gems of information.

ME IN A HAT!

This is based on a game called 'Fear in a hat'. Each member of the group writes down on a piece of paper four things about themselves:

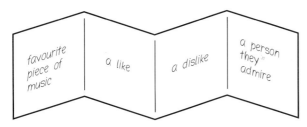

These are then folded and placed in a hat (or the bin) and everyone takes one out. Members take turns to read out their list and says who they think it is and why. This gives good feedback as to how others perceive us. The list of categories is endless and the game itself is easily adapted for any stage of a group. The categories can be quite innocuous, such as favourite colour, or more revealing, as with 'one thing about me I'd like to change', 'one of my best points' or 'one of my worst points'.

A BIG WIN

Each member in turn describes what they would do if they won a lot of money and why.

WHO AM I?

This is a more active game, getting members walking about and talking to each other. Each member has a label attached to their back, so that they cannot see it. On the label is written the name of a famous person or character from fiction. Examples might be Mickey Mouse, Margaret Thatcher, Batman, Winston Churchill, Greta Garbo — the list is endless. You can have sports personalities, royalty, film stars, politicians, people from history, musicians, comedians and so on.

The idea is that group members go around trying to find out who they are, but they cannot say "Who am I?" They must deduce their identity by a process of elimination: for example, "Am I a woman?" "Am I an actress?"

This doesn't usually take too long and is good fun. It usually ends up with just one member left unidentified and the rest frantically trying to give them clues.

At a later stage in the group when sufficient trust and understanding has been developed it is possible to take this one step further.

Merely substitute fictional names for the names of group members. One sly trick is to give a couple of them their own names. Again this provides good feedback about how others perceive us.

WHO ARE WE?

This is much the same as 'Who am I?' but, having found your own identity, you have to team up with your partner, for example Batman and Robin, Fred Astaire and Ginger Rogers.

ON BEING OLD

The group sits in a close circle and we go around saying how we feel about how old we are and what relevance age has, if any.

Brainstorm a list of the qualities we associate with youth, then locate those or comparable qualities in ourselves.

Then go on to use the *Oxford Book of Ages* (Sampson, 1988), which is full of quotations for every age from one to a hundred. Discuss the quotations and how we feel about them. Do we agree, do they make us angry or make us laugh? This can be a very enlightening group but needs careful direction if members are to gain from it; thinking about how old we are can be quite a saddening experience but at the same time gives us a perspective on our lives.

CHANGES

Have the group get into pairs and stand facing each other. One of each pair then turns around whilst the other quickly changes one thing about their appearance. When ready ask the others to turn back and try to recognize what change has occurred. This is often much harder than it sounds (eg. earrings removed). When everyone has discovered the change switch roles and repeat.

MAGIC BOX

Sitting in a circle, describe to the group a large imaginary box in the middle of the circle, then ask them to imagine an object that might be in that box. Allow a few minutes for this. Then ask each member in turn to go into the middle and mime removing the object from the box and using it. The group then has to decide what it is. Alternatively give the members each a piece of paper naming the item they will have to mime.

BLIND QUOTE

With the group in a fairly wide circle this time and a chair in the middle ask for a volunteer and sit them on the chair. Blindfold them and ask the rest of the group to walk around the room and then sit down again in different chairs. Give one of the group members a small quote to read; then the person in the chair has to guess who read it.

ONLY POLITICS

Using a blackboard ask the group members to brainstorm a list of political parties. Here are some examples: Conservative, Labour, Liberal Democrat, Communist, Green Party, Scottish Nationalist, Welsh Nationalist, Ulster Unionist, Sinn Fein, National Front, Socialist Workers Party, Silly Party, Democratic Party, Republican Party; there are many others.

Then briefly discuss the relative merits of each and pronounce a general election. Give out pens and paper and ask each member to select who they would vote for by writing it down. Fold up the papers and throw them in the bin. Then proceed to count the votes by marking ticks on the blackboard as you fish each vote out of the bin.

This often leads to heated debate, usually focusing on personalities such as party leaders, and it is interesting to discuss what qualities of leadership the group thinks various people exhibit.

To focus this a little you could ask them to choose one person they feel would be a good choice to run the country, for argument's sake, as leader of a coalition or as a president.

My own choice would be Guy Fawkes . . . the only person to enter parliament with honest intentions.

"WE'LL ALL GO TOGETHER WHEN WE GO!"

This is an update on an old game which involved throwing people from a hot air balloon. It is not for the squeamish. The old game described a hot air balloon journey which got into difficulties and the only way of saving four of the five people in it was for one to make the ultimate sacrifice or, failing that, be thrown overboard. In our version, someone, somewhere has pressed 'the' button and full-scale nuclear war has broken out. However five fortunate people have managed to get into the protective bunker just in time. So in order to start the game, ask the group to choose five famous people, it can be anybody, or five occupations. Then describe in detail the nuclear scenario.

The bunker has developed a leak. Radiation at dangerous levels is seeping in and you must move to an adjacent bunker. There are however only four radiation suits with which to make the transition safely and they can only be used once. You are forced into the position of having to argue who gets a radiation suit. There are two ways to do this. Firstly, the group can decide between themselves who, or which occupation, is least necessary, and arrive at a mutual decision. Secondly, group members have to adopt identities or occupations and argue for their own survival.

DRAW THIS

Have prepared several pieces of paper with abstract drawings on, for example as in Figure 1.

Give one member one of these drawings and give the rest pieces of paper and pencils. The person with the drawing then describes it to the rest, who must each draw their version according to their interpretation of the description. Usually the variations at the end are far and wide and this illustrates how we all perceive the same reality in different ways.

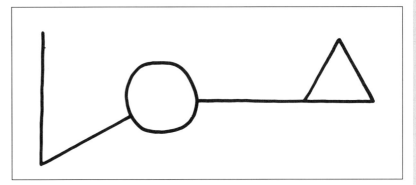

Figure 1 *Draw This*

CHARADES

This is also known as 'give us a clue' (since a TV programme). It is a good lighthearted game for the early stages of a group, which can be varied enormously. Group members mime the words to songs, films, TV shows and so on, and the others must try to guess the answer.

WHO IS IT?

This is a version of 'twenty questions'. One member decides upon a famous character or person, the others have to guess it by

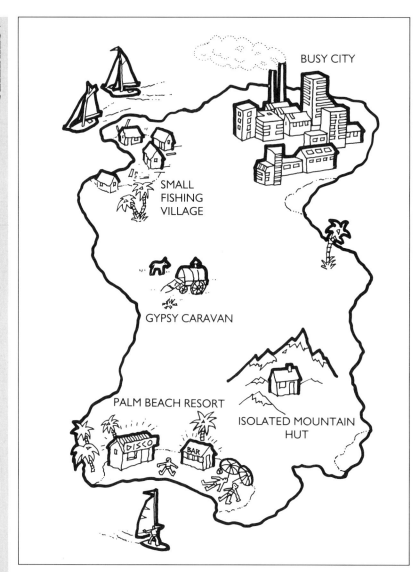

Figure 2 *Island*

asking questions: for instance, "Woman or man?" "Is it a cartoon character?" Set a limit of twenty questions if you like.

A useful variation of this is to ask 'it' to think of another group member, with the rest trying to guess who it is.

CHINESE WHISPERS

Write on a piece of paper a message to be passed verbally around the group. The last one writes it down and then the group compares the two versions. Explain that you can only say the message once and that you must whisper it when you pass it on.

ISLAND

Draw on a blackboard an island including:

1 a busy city
2 a small fishing village
3 a busy palm beach holiday resort
4 an isolated mountain hut
5 a gypsy caravan.
    (See Figure 2)

Describe each of the five areas in some detail, emphasizing for example the bustle of the city, availability of shops, goods and entertainment. Similarly for the small fishing village, detail the quiet, and how everybody knows everybody and you cannot do anything without the whole village knowing about it. When you have described all five areas each member of the group must say where they would choose to live and why. This says a lot about the kind of person we are and the ensuing discussion can focus on aspects such as how much we need other people around us, loneliness, life in the city and so on.

ACTIVITIES

DESERT ISLAND DISCS

This is fairly self-explanatory, being based on a popular British radio programme. We just expand it a little and include several variations:

1 Ask each member of the group to imagine life on a desert island and get them to decide upon a book, a piece of music and a treasured possession which they would like to have with them.

2 Who you would like to be marooned with and why:

"a ravishing beauty skilled in the art of distilling the finest liquor from any spare plants who . . ." I digress!

3 A useful variation is to get members to write on a piece of paper a book, piece of music, treasured object and hero with whom they would want to be marooned. Fold the papers, place in a hat, pass it around, pick one out then guess who it is and say why.

HOW I SEE MYSELF!

This is similar to 'If they were a flower'. Get the members to write on a piece of paper how they see themselves as, for example, a colour, piece of music, animal, plant, food, means of transport. Choose only four. Fold the papers, place in the bin, pick one out, guess who and say why.

"IT'S A LIVING"

This game stimulates lively discussion as to the relative importance or otherwise of various occupations. The grading list below is taken from Graham Sargeant's *A Textbook of Sociology* and is a so-called 'normal' ranking in order of importance (reading across):

◆ Medical officer of health   ◆ Company director

◆ Chartered accountant   ◆ Solicitor
◆ Business manager   ◆ Works manager
◆ Farmer   ◆ Nonconformist minister
◆ Civil servant   ◆ Jobbing master builder
◆ Elementary school teacher   ◆ News reporter
◆ Chef   ◆ Coal miner
◆ Fitter   ◆ Policeman
◆ Carpenter   ◆ Bricklayer
◆ Commercial traveller   ◆ Insurance agent
◆ Newsagent and tobacconist ◆ Routine clerk
◆ Tractor driver   ◆ Dock labourer
◆ Agricultural labourer   ◆ Shop assistant
◆ Carter   ◆ Railway porter
◆ Barman   ◆ Road sweeper

Use this grading to generate a good group discussion.

Write the list in random order on the blackboard. I usually find it best to choose just a dozen occupations which vary widely, otherwise it tends to take too long. Then ask the group to grade them in order of importance by placing a number 1 to 12 against each one, discussing their merits or otherwise along the way.

When you have arrived at a ranking with what could loosely be regarded as consensus inform the group that, following a nuclear war or a shipwreck on a desert island, there will only be six survivors. Who would you want with you on a desert island or in a hostile environment?

This usually upsets the previous order of importance . . . could I interest you in an insurance policy?

TRIALS

The group is a jury.

You can either get a case out of a paper, national or local, where you know the outcome, or you can invent a scenario of your own which you should describe in some detail. The group should then be asked to arrive at a verdict and deliver a sentence.

Examples could be:

1   someone caught speeding on the way to hospital with an expectant wife
2   a man on unemployment benefit caught shoplifting
3   a company boss fiddling his tax returns.

A useful adjunct to further discussions relating to the difficulty of sentencing and whether punishments work would be to brainstorm various crimes and then allot sentences.

GROUP LINES

Ask the members to stand in a line according to:

1   height — small to tall
2   birthdays — January to December
3   politics — left to right
4   introvert to extrovert
5   age

and so on. This is a good warm-up but also lets us know something about our fellow group members.

BURIED IN THE SAND

There is a great disaster impending and it is likely that all life on earth will be wiped out. There is a small chance that life exists on another planet and sometime in the future a being may land on the remains of our planet.

You have a small lead chest into which you can place several items which you feel depict the kind of people we were.

You can let the group decide on their own or you can prompt by choosing categories, such as book, machine, record, antique.

CURRENT AFFAIRS

This is a good non-threatening way of drawing people in as a discussion group by asking their opinions. It can highlight cognitive deficits and can elsewhere provide the basis for a reminiscence session.

It can be done in many ways, as previously in 'What the papers say' from the 'Warm-ups' section, or you can study the paper beforehand and pick out issues to read to the group for comment and discussion. Try to find opposing viewpoints and contentious issues and balance them with more lighthearted snippets.

Alternatively you can let the members choose the articles and issues by giving them some papers fifteen minutes before. It is useful to give them coloured marker pens so that they can mark the appropriate place. For a more complicated current affairs group, see 'Parole' and its variations.

THE COMMON GALAXY

Many years hence life has been discovered on many new planets which have co-existed in harmony for many of our earth years. They have joined together to form a 'common galaxy' and now for its own protection earth is seeking to join this group. It has sent its ambassadors to plead its case in front of the common galaxy new entrants' committee. Divide the group into two:

Group 1: must put forward evidence as to why earth should be allowed to join

Group 2: should put the case against.

PAROLE

Select at random twenty famous people — either from history or from the present. Brainstorm the names or use newspapers, getting the members to shout out the names.

Write them down on the blackboard as they are called out.

Inform the group that all these people are in prison and are now up for parole. Their original crimes are not taken into account and unfortunately only six of them can be given parole . . . who and why?

A useful variation is to do a current affairs group using the day's papers and as you go through them list twenty people, famous or otherwise, who have been mentioned. When you have finished discussing the news, look again at the twenty names on the blackboard and ask the group to decide which ten would be most useful in a tricky situation, such as being marooned on an island, in a lifeboat, in a spaceship, on a voyage around the world lasting a year, which ten would form a good government and so on. What qualities would you look for in someone with whom you would be spending so much time within a confined space?

Other ideas for following through the current affairs debate, having culled a dozen or so names from the paper are:

1 Leaders
  What qualities are needed?
  Who would we choose?
  Rank them in order.

2 Stuck on a boat for a year
  What would you look for in a person with whom you have got to be cooped up for a year?
  Rank them.

3 Counselling
  What qualities are needed?
  Who could you share a problem with from the given list?

4 Used cars
  What are the qualities of a good salesman?
  From whom on your list would you buy a used car?

LEADERSHIP

This is a useful group for stimulating debate and good healthy argument. Give each member a piece of paper with the following qualities which are often associated with leadership:

- fairness
- ruthlessness
- intelligence
- background
- resourcefulness
- fitness
- consistency
- loyalty
- kindness
- good listener

- understanding
- honesty
- appearance
- courage
- maturity
- determination
- public speaking
- enthusiasm
- decisiveness
- unselfishness

Then ask them to rank them 1 to 20, placing a 1 against the quality they feel is most important and 20 against that which they feel is least important.

When everyone has finished go through each quality in turn, discussing why each feels it to be important or not. This can get very interesting: we spent ages once just discussing what maturity was. Do you gain it, do you slip in and out of it, has it got anything at all to do with age?

The debate and argument can be further enhanced by asking for examples of good leaders. You can throw in a few contentious examples such as Arthur Scargill, Caesar, Churchill, Reagan, de Gaulle, Chairman Mao. What was it about these people that made people follow them? You might hate everything they stood for, but were they still good leaders?

This is obviously a good group to bring out at election times both at home and abroad. We used it when Margaret Thatcher resigned. The diversity of opinion regarding her qualities and views was fuel for much disagreement, very healthy and very frustrating. You must keep your own political bias at a non-influential level.

QUESTIONS

Each member is given a piece of paper and a pencil and asked to write down a question. The pieces of paper are then folded several times and tossed into the waste paper bin. Each member then takes out one of the folded pieces of paper. Nominate someone to start and go around reading out each question and commenting on it. This is good because it is anonymous (if members want it to be) and because its depth is entirely at the control of the group members.

The leader must judge the mood and coherence of the group in order to know how far to explore each question. Examples of questions that have come up in our groups are:

◆ How long will I have to come here?

◆ What's the weather like in the south of France?

The range varies, according to the group's status, from irrelevant and glib, to currently topical and deeply personal. Because of this, and the exercise's easiness, it is one that is well worth repeating regularly.

BABY FACE

Ask each member to bring in old photos of themselves as babies and youngsters, or school children. Throw them all in the bin and pass it around. The rest is obvious — who is it? This is good fun and leads to much reminiscing. Don't forget to include yourself — ahh, isn't he cute!

DEAR MARJIE

Read out the problems from the 'problem' page of a daily newspaper or women's magazine and ask the group to come up with a reply as to what the person should do and why. This can be a lighthearted session or can be adapted for use as a cognitive or support group session. By writing the problems yourself you can focus on issues which may be being avoided by group members.

CHARACTERIZED

This is a very stimulating group and can be used over several weeks looking at different areas. Basically it looks at stereotyping and explores attitudes toward different groups within society. First choose your target group(s), for example elderly people, youth, northerners, southerners, English people, foreigners, the group members themselves, Conservatives, Socialists, Republicans, Democrats, men, women.

Then draw a grid on a blackboard or flipchart ten squares by ten. Along the top, brainstorm ten characteristics of humans (or supply them yourselves with careful preparation). Down the left, brainstorm ten characters from your chosen target group(s). The characters do not all have to be real: you can use fictional characters as these often have much influence over attitude formation. Examples in the elderly age group are Corporal Jones (Clive Dunn) from 'Dad's Army', Scrooge, Father Christmas, Miss Haversham, Alf Garnett. Don't have too many fictional characters though.

Then merely tick which characteristics these characters indicate to the group members.

When you have filled in the grid you will have a focus for discussion on why you have allotted certain characteristics to certain people and not to others. It is useful if you have opposing characters, for instance five men, five women, or five elderly people, five young people, so that you can highlight and discuss the differences you have given to the characters. This leads naturally on to discussion about stereotyping and what factors influence our attitudes to various people.

A useful variant for elderly people's groups is to discuss youth and choose ten characteristics of it. These are then plotted against ten elderly characters or people of the group's choosing. It usually shows us that the characteristics of youth are still existent in old age.

Examples of some characteristics and their opposites:

careful	careless
humorous	solemn
lazy	hardworking
courageous	timid
slow	quick-witted
challenging	accepting

happy	sad
talkative	quiet
leading	following
outgoing	shy
co-operative	unco-operative
forgiving	unforgiving
emotional	unemotional
polite	impolite
deceitful	truthful
stubborn	yielding
popular	unpopular
quick-tempered	easy-going
considerate	inconsiderate
kind	unkind
suspicious	trusting
intolerant	tolerant
unsympathetic	sympathetic
highly-strung	calm
straightforward	devious
pessimistic	optimistic
aggressive	passive
reliable	unreliable
modest	immodest

PAY ATTENTION — I'LL BE ASKING QUESTIONS

This is a variation on 'Changes'. Here you split your group up into two lines facing each other, and ask them to take a good long hard look at their opposite partner.

Then sit them down back to back and have them fill in the following questionnaire:

1 How old do you guess they are (be careful as this could lead to blows)?

2 What is the colour and style of their hair?

3 Do they weigh more than you?

4 Are they taller than you?

5 What colour eyes do they have?

6 Are they wearing any jewellery?

7 Describe their dress, including shoes

8 Describe their face

9 Name one distinguishing feature

10 If you had to give them a nickname what would it be?

Obviously this can be lengthened, for example by using 'If they were a flower' type questions. It is usually great fun.

Another variation which you can slip into any group is to have a similar preprinted questionnaire which focuses only on appearance and arrange for one of your friends to interrupt a group, borrow some chalk, ask you a question, pick up a book, or just breeze in and say "Oh, I'm sorry!" and walk out again. Then at the end of the group give out the questionnaire to test their powers of observation, for instance with questions on height, hair, clothes, the time they interrupted, whether their jumper was acrylic, nylon or wool, what was the 'sell by' date on the packet of biscuits they were carrying . . . keep it easy!

PUT YOUR HANDS IN THIS BAG — TRUST ME!

This is really a perception game but it is included here because it also tests our powers of communication and description and it can be very good fun. Basically you gather together a number of unusual items and put each in a pillow case. Choose a victim and ask them to put their hands behind their back and into the pillow case. They must then describe the object to the rest of the group who must decide what it is. This provides a wonderful opportunity to group leaders with a wicked sense of humour. Half a pound of pork sausages spring to mind! Maybe a ferret or two!

IT'S YOURS

Ask each member to bring in an object or personal item of their choice and get them to give it to you earlier when nobody else is looking. They should just be small things like jewellery, something they carry around with them, a lighter, a charm, something they like, such as a tape, book, an item of clothing, a picture.

Then in the group place them all on a table and ask each member to pick one up, ensuring that it is not theirs.

Then ask each member to say whose they think it is and why. If they guess wrong the group chips in.

IT IS I (IN A HAT)!

This is a variation on 'Fear in a hat'. Get everyone to write down one thing that they think is characteristic of them, fold it up and throw it in the bin. Pass the bin around, with each taking a piece of paper. Go around and say who you think it is and why. Unless you are in a deeply therapeutic group you should insist that the characteristics are positive: fun-loving, patient, kind, as opposed to irritable, stubborn, etc. If however you feel your group can give positive feedback to negative self-descriptions you could focus on these qualities and explore others' perceptions of individual self-assessments.

WHAT PRICE IS IT?

What you need here are large pictures from magazines of items of shopping, clothes, hardware, food, cigarettes, drinks and so on.

These are then held up and the price is asked: "What would you pay for this?" Try to get a current price, for example a supermarket receipt. The prices often surprise people who frequently have not done much shopping for a while, relying on relatives or home helps.

The prices can be compared with yesteryear and relative values can be discussed. Is it worth all that money? What is a luxury and what is a necessity?

A trip around the local supermarket or shopping centre is usually an eye opener; things have changed drastically in the last few years. We never used to need fabric softeners, and what is a fridge deodorizer?

ANTIQUES ROADSHOW

This is self-explanatory and is based on the television series with which most people will be familiar. Simply get together five or so antique items and one at a time pass them around the group to decide what they are, how old they are and how much they think they are worth. It does not matter if you do not know their exact value; it is interesting to see and discuss how people value things differently.

An alternative is to cut out pictures of antiques and pass these around, but having the object there is much better. There is also a quiz game based on the 'Antiques Roadshow' which can be useful. Another good book is the *Observer's Book of Victoriana*, or an old copy of *Miller's Antiques Guide*.

These groups are designed to help us to explore how we see ourselves and how others see us. By definition they are groups which concentrate on cognition. The dictionary tells us that this is the faculty of knowing and perceiving. It is what we believe, in this case, about ourselves. The groups focus on what we think, feel and believe and contrast this with the opinion of others and observable 'facts' about ourselves.

I am indebted to Aaron T Beck and Ruth L Greenberg for their work in this field in giving a clear understanding of the concepts involved and would recommend *Coping with Depression* (1974) to anyone who wants to know more.

Cognitive therapy is a valuable therapy for people who are depressed or those whose self-esteem is low. Shy, introverted people and those whose social skills are deficient because of a poor self-concept can also be helped.

We think about ourselves differently when depressed. As a result we act differently. Commonly we end up with a low opinion of our own self-worth and abilities. We become apathetic and withdrawn and, above all, gloomy in our outlook. This becomes the reality for us. Depression makes us think we deserve such a bleak existence. It makes us believe we are worthless and unworthy of help. In extreme cases we feel unworthy of even continuing our existence and we attempt to curtail it.

Such negative thoughts are commonplace amongst depressed people and as a result their feelings are correspondingly negative: "I think I am worthless, therefore I feel sad."

Cognitive therapy aims to challenge what the individual thinks; it sees negative thoughts as errors of judgement, caused by the depression, which rapidly become self-fulfilling prophecies.

Similarly if you don't practise social skills you quickly come to believe you have none and subsequently lose much of your self-esteem.

Thus in depression many of your bad feelings are based on mistakes of thinking or altered thinking.

However, in depression we still retain our intellectual capabilities even though we may not think we do, and cognitive therapy hinges on this fact.

What we can do is to try and recognize our negative thoughts and try to substitute more realistic ones. This is where groupwork is so useful as we can have our negative opinions rejected by others and more positive qualities reinforced.

We shall concentrate here on three activities: an incomplete sentences exercise, a self inventory and a social skills checklist. They are useful for exploring how we feel about ourselves and form the nucleus of a groupwork programme which aims to redevelop our positive self-esteem. The three tools focus on how people interact in social situations, that is, being with other people and talking to them and so on. They help to highlight particular difficulties that we may have in these situations. They help us to explore what makes us feel anxious and uncomfortable. Having identified this much we can then go on to explore and practice strategies and alternative ways of coping. The three tools give us a statement of how we see ourselves which can then be contrasted with how others perceive us, and our actual performance in our daily lives. As a result, we can open our own perceptions to the scrutiny of others. It is useful to focus in some depth upon our assumed deficits. The tools force us to explore our beliefs in detail and identify specific difficulties; this in itself is beneficial as it helps us to move away from a feeling of holistic inadequacy or generalized worthlessness. This is reinforced by support from the group and indeed positive reinforcement by others in the group is the prime factor in achieving lasting change.

The therapist and the group can show us how negative thoughts tend to be 'automatic'. They are not arrived at by logic. They stem from the low opinion of ourselves depression inflicts upon us.

If negative thoughts are logically examined by self-analysis and the opinion of others they can be shown to be unreasonable and we can start to see how they get in the way of our lives.

We can recognize that in depression we don't question these thoughts, we hopelessly accept them as being perfectly plausible. The longer you are in this vicious spiral the deeper you sink.

In a specific group situation we can be exposed to positive reinforcement so that we have the chance to break out of the spiral of gloom. Recognizing negative thoughts and coming to understand the part they play in our illness is therefore crucial to our recovery.

Some typical errors of thinking which can be explored using the incomplete sentences, social skills checklist and self inventory are:

1 **Exaggeration:**
Small difficulties become disasters, problems become catastrophes. While exaggerating the difficulty we also correspondingly underestimate our ability to deal with it and jump to gloomy conclusions.

2 **Overgeneralizing:**
We make broad sweeping statements, for example, "I'm hopeless", "I'm a complete and utter failure."

3 **Ignoring the positive**
We tend to remember only the bad things.

The aim of cognitive therapy then is to help us to identify and correct unrealistic thinking, caused by depression, which brings us to erroneous conclusions about ourselves, thus giving us feelings of worthlessness and all its associated apathetic behaviour.

If the group puts this information across and reinforces positive aspects with mutual support then something worthwhile has been achieved. The greater the group cohesiveness and identity accomplished, the stronger become the messages put across. Peer support from a well estalished group has a very strong influence.

The facilitator of such a group should regard their position as a great privilege and recognize the power of the group dynamics which are at work.

Many of the interaction games can be used here as well to build cohesiveness. They can be directed to highlight how we feel about ourselves and how others see us.

Interaction within the group can highlight significant relationships in the clients' lives. Changes experienced in this setting and social skills practised in the group can be carried over into ways of relating to people in the outside world. The group cohesion provides a safe arena for practising such skills.

It is important that in these groups the therapists are not changed, as this will destroy cohesiveness and inhibit participation.

Cognitive therapy is also useful for those groups whose members have common problems or circumstances. They can help us to look in depth at our perception of ourselves and how we deal with particular problems or situations, for example, following bereavement, living alone and following discharge from hospital.

In the latter case the group should begin well before discharge so that a powerful support mechanism is set up early on.

This will help alleviate fears of isolation and such thoughts as "Will I be able to cope?"

Merely knowing that the group will continue after discharge is a great comfort and source of strength in itself. Indeed this applies to many social groups, the membership of which is a great source of support and positive reinforcement to us all.

The three main sources of material for the groupwork sessions are, then:

1 Incomplete sentences
2 Self inventories
3 Social skills checklist

These can be used in a large variety of ways as the basis of a group discussion and self-exploration.

It is impossible to dictate how they should be used, that is for you to decide with your group's needs in mind. It depends on what stage the group is at and what particular issues, skills or concepts are pertinent to your group.

You can vary your approach accordingly and pick a few items to concentrate on each week, or design your own checklists for group members to fill in and thereby draw profiles of how they see themselves. I would suggest you use a little of each.

INCOMPLETE SENTENCES

One thing I've always wanted to do is . . .

Something I could change now is . . .

In this group I feel . . .

One thing that really irritates me is . . .

It worries me that . . .

I get angry when . . .

I get depressed when . . .

My main problem is . . .

My biggest weakness is . . .

My greatest strength is . . .

The best thing I've ever done is . . .

One thing that embarrasses me is . . .

The most important thing in my life is . . .

I dislike . . .

I like . . .

ACTIVITIES

Something I could change this week is . . .

A change I'd like to make but don't think I can is . . .

I trust people who . . .

One thing about me that people might be surprised to know is . . .

I distrust people who . . .

I feel happy when . . .

I wish I could . . .

I can never . . .

I used to . . .

One thing I really enjoy is . . .

My goal for this week is . . .

The worst thing I've ever done is . . .

One good thing that happened this week was . . .

My greatest joy is . . .

The last time I lost my temper was . . .

One thing I'm good at is . . .

A person I really admire is . . .

The hardest thing I've ever done is . . .

People think I'm . . .

The best thing about me is . . .

If I could change one thing about me it would be . . .

It would be easy for me to . . .

Obviously there are many more you can think of. Each one of these sentences says a great deal about ourselves. You can use just one sentence for each group if you want, or use contrasting sentences. You can vary the amount of self-disclosure and anonymity according to the needs and stage of the group. Obviously you start with fairly innocuous ones that are not very

personal or disclosing and gradually explore further. You could do a round of saying the sentences or get members to write them down and put them in our old friend the hat. Members then read out someone else's and each discusses what it tells them about that person. They could paraphrase them, saying what they feel that person is trying to say and how they think that person might feel about it. This will give good feedback.

There is no need to identify who they think it is, but if the group is strong enough this will allow for more feedback from the rest of the group.

SELF INVENTORY

Here we describe where we feel we belong on a continuum between contrasting qualities. The aim as always is to foster positive self-image by inducing positive feedback from our peers and hence to increase self-knowledge. The continua are:

Co-operative	Unco-operative
Emotional	Unemotional
Deceitful	Truthful
Popular	Unpopular
Careful	Careless
Lazy	Hardworking
Challenging	Accepting
Talkative	Quiet
Kind	Unkind
Intolerant	Tolerant
Highly-strung	Calm
Humorous	Solemn
Slow	Quick-witted

Leading	Following
Outgoing	Shy
Forgiving	Unforgiving
Polite	Impolite
Stubborn	Yielding
Quick-tempered	Easy-going
Considerate	Inconsiderate
Suspicious	Trusting
Unsympathetic	Sympathetic
Go-ahead	Cautious
Straightforward	Devious
Pessimistic	Optimistic
Aggressive	Passive
Reliable	Non-dependable
Modest	Immodest
Successful	Inadequate

The list is obviously not exhaustive and you can add qualities you feel need exploring by your clients.

It is important that the group leader directs the group towards and focuses on feedback. Merely getting everyone to say where they lie on the continuum is of little value if it is not explored.

You can express these qualities singly or you can have them as a chart to be filled in and then discussed.

This would have each quality displayed thus:

OUTGOING 3   2   1   0   1   2   3 **SHY**

Ask the members to work through the sheet in their own time, putting a circle around where they think they fit.

Sheets can be produced at subsequent sessions and worked through.

Another useful variant using the same format, but slightly more complicated, uses the concept of Johari's Window (see page 34), which we will explore later.

In this variation we think of:

1 How we see ourselves — ○
2 How we think others see us — △
3 How we would like to be — □

We use the same 3 2 1 0 1 2 3 continuum and place the symbols along it where we feel appropriate; thus, for me:

OUTGOING 3 □②△ 1   0   1   2   3 **SHY**

Again the key is to use these as you feel appropriate.

SOCIAL SKILLS CHECKLIST

This is a list of situations in which people may or may not have difficulty.

Again you can add to it situations which are pertinent to your group members. They are in no particular order and you can either go through a few each week or ask members of the group to work through them outside the group, commenting on their relative degree of difficulty.

1 Eating or drinking with others
2 Going into local newsagents
3 Going into a supermarket

ACTIVITIES

4 Walking alone down the street

5 Going around town on a Saturday afternoon

6 Being looked at

7 Using public transport

8 Talking to people in authority

9 Going into a crowded room

10 Going into a pub

11 Taking things back to a shop if they are faulty

12 Going to a party

13 Going to the cinema or theatre

14 Talking to strangers

15 Asking for help

16 Going for an interview

17 Expressing your anger

18 Talking about yourself

19 Saying no

20 Standing or sitting close to someone else

21 Making friends

22 Talking to someone of the opposite sex

23 Making decisions for yourself

24 Making decisions for others

25 Eating out in restaurants and cafes

26 Initiating conversation

27 Answering the telephone

28 Answering the door

29 Disagreeing with people and letting them know

30 Making eye contact

31 Complaining.

Following completion, members can compare responses and obtain feedback as to how others felt about their responses.

One variant which helps elicit feedback is to bring out the hat again. Members write, for example, a sentence completing "One thing I can't do" or "I feel uneasy about" and one "I can do" or "I feel relaxed about".

This gives immediate feedback, such as "I think this is Danny because I know he can go into pubs, but he says restaurants are a problem for him." The rest of the group can then chip in their therapeutic ten pennyworth.

This can help people to explore common fears and look at what factors are in play which elicit fear in which particular situations.

The use of role play is advantageous here, enabling scenarios to be acted out in the relative comfort of the group. Introverted members can be asked to play arrogant types who are very out-going to explore how it feels. Skills practised in safety can then be gradually practised in a real setting by the client.

It is useful to set weekly goals and ask people to write down their feelings immediately after their tasks for discussion at the next group.

There are other exercises which are useful for this type of group. They can be used in a variety of ways at various stages in the development of the group.

FEAR IN A HAT

This uses the incomplete sentences, with the therapist directing the aim of the group and its particular focus. Members are asked to write down one sentence of the type, I wish, I fear, I hope, I feel, I think, I believe.

The therapist can then focus this on a chosen situation or use the exercise in each session to focus upon how people feel during each session.

Members take one sentence each from the hat and paraphrase it, for example, "I think that this person is saying that . . ."

The group can comment on this interpretation and many interpretations could follow. They all give feedback to the anonymous (or otherwise) writer that we share and understand how they feel, thereby reducing feelings of isolation.

TRANSACTIONAL ANALYSIS

Throughout my early meetings with transactional analysis I always felt, and still do to some degree, that it leaves a lot to be desired.

I felt it was far too simplistic a concept. However simple is often best, and it can provide a useful way of examining how we see ourselves and how others see us. It is another method of categorizing ourselves and in doing so it, much like the other exercises, helps us to be more specific about our difficulties and moves us away from generalized gloom. This process, of forcing us to highlight specific details of our self-perception, facilitates greater feedback from our peers. Thus we are not using transactional analysis as a specific means of achieving change but merely as a tool for examining our self-perceptions. We are encouraged, as practitioners, to reflect upon our practice. Transactional analysis helps us to reflect upon our behaviour and perceptions of others.

Basically it identifies what it calls five ego states and their associated qualities:

1 **Critical Parent** critical, demanding, "What will people say?", irritable, obeying rules

2 **Free Child** fun-loving, encouraging, immediacy, must have it now, curious, innocent

3 **Adult** rational, decision maker, correctness, weigh up pros and cons, confident, calm

4 **Nurturing Parent** caring, loving, approving, concerned, sympathetic

5 **Adaptive Child** feeling sorry for ourselves, "I can't do it", willing to please, worried, sulking, not my fault.

This is only a rough sketch but it is enough to try and get group members to put themselves in one of the five categories. Members can explore the categories and discuss the qualities therein, good and bad. Where would the qualities they identified in the self inventory place them as an ego state?

JOHARI'S WINDOW

Again this is only a rough sketch and for further elaboration I would point you to S J Sundeen *et al* (CV Mosby, 1976), *Nurse, Client, Interaction*.

Johari divided the 'person' into four squares of a window:

1 What is known about us to ourselves and to others

2 What is known about us only to ourselves

3 What is known about us only to others

4 What is known neither by self nor others.

This last one is a difficult concept: if we do not know it and nobody else does, then can it really exist?

The other three categories are fairly sound, however, and we can try and get group members and ourselves to identify certain aspects of our personality and behaviour which fit those categories. Like transactional analysis, Johari's Window helps us to explore the way we feel about ourselves and thus provide the opportunity for others to provide feedback. We hear much about self-examination for breast cancer and other physical conditions, but little upon health promotion techniques for mental illness.

GOAL PLANNING

Planning goals, however small, is a good way of identifying what steps to take next and the group can help us with this process.

The following can be used:

One thing I hope to achieve this week . . .

This week I will try and . . .

I hope this week to be able to . . .

Invent your own and get members to write them down and give them to you.

Next week read them out in turn and get members to talk through their attempts. Non-achievement must be regarded as a brave attempt and difficulties explored in full in the group.

OTHER IDEAS

Other interaction games which we described earlier can also be useful here:

◆ If they were a flower

◆ Island

◆ Desert island discs

◆ How I see myself

◆ Under a fiver

◆ Group lines – on a more personal theme

◆ Buried in the sand – six things about me

◆ Who I am – using group members

The idea behind this group is to look at how we feel about how old we are. Have an open round of saying how old we are and whether we like that age or feel sad about our passing years. We look back at what we feel was our favourite age and forwards to what we hope for our years to come.

A useful way of focusing the discussion is to use quotations, sayings and poetry. A good source is the *Oxford Book of Ages* (Sampson, 1988) which is full of quotes and small passages relating to each year from one to a hundred. With this you can read a few from everyone's age. One word of warning. It seems that the great majority of the quotes are rather gloomy: avoid these and focus on those which highlight the positive qualities of later life.

You will find many poems relating to the ageing process, for example:

Ted Hughes, *Old Age gets up*; *Retired colonel*

Philip Larkin, *The old fool*; *Mrs Bleaney*

Roy Fuller, *Consolations*

These can often focus our feelings more acutely than a small quote.

However, here are a few tasters:

'You are as old as you feel'
Anon

'Tomorrow I will haul down the flag of hypocrisy,
I will devote my grey hairs to wine.
My life's span has reached 70,
If I don't enjoy myself now, when shall I?'
From 12th century Rubaiyat of Omar Khayyam

'In July when I bury my nose in a hazel bush, I feel 15 years old again'
Corot, 1867

'There's many a good tune played on an old fiddle'
Samuel Butler

'To me old age is always 15 years older than I am'
B Baruch

'I have always lived an unhealthy life . . .
All the doctors who wanted to forbid me to smoke and drink are dead. But I am quietly going on living'
Sibelius, aged 87 (1972)

'What I wouldn't give to be 70 again'
O W Holmes, aged 91, on seeing a pretty girl

'If I'd known I was going to live this long,
I'd have taken better care of myself'
Eubie Blake, jazz pianist, aged 99

Ronald Blythe's book, *The View in Winter*, is another source of good views about old age and ageing.

Focusing on our age enables us to take stock of where we are in our lives and the therapist's task is to allow us to ventilate our fears without becoming over gloomy. It provides us with a chance to set goals for the future and look at our positive qualities. Having done this we can look to and discuss how best to use our retirement years.

Simulation games are great fun, but demand a large degree of awareness and co-operation. However you can vary them according to your needs, making them as easy or as difficult as you wish and indeed inventing your own.

Basically they involve describing a scenario in which a group of people are faced with a series of choices in difficult or awkward situations. They are given certain information and a list of articles and have to decide how to get themselves out of the mess in which they find themselves! It is useful to try and make it as realistic as possible by providing some props: for example, in a mountain snow storm, drape a few sheets into a snow cave and sit your group in it with a few props such as an ice axe, box of matches, whistle, torch, bar of Kendal Mint Cake, rope, map.

These exercises can be done by individual members of the group, but it is far better to get some interaction going by splitting your group into two smaller ones of, say, four each and then comparing their different responses to the situation afterwards.

LOST IN SPACE

Having got your two groups huddled together in the wreck of their space craft and surrounded by moonlike props you can begin to unfold their plight. Tell them they are in a space craft (or what is left of it) on the light side of the moon. Mechanical difficulties caused you to crash-land 200 miles away from the rendezvous point with your mother ship. The crash smashed most of your supplies but you are left with:

a box of matches

food concentrate

50 foot of nylon rope

parachute silk

portable heating unit

two .45 calibre pistols

one case of dehydrated milk

two 100 pound oxygen tanks

a map of the moon's surface

inflatable life raft

magnetic compass

five gallons of water

signal flares

first aid kit

solar power receiver/transmitter.

(Give each person a copy of this list and a pencil.)

Now tell them that their survival depends upon reaching the mother ship; if they take the wrong things they won't make it. Rank the fifteen items in order of importance, placing a number 1 against the most important and a 15 against the least important.

Now give them between 15 and 30 minutes to do this; keep going between the groups to see how they are doing and to chivvy them along.

When they have finished, let each group describe how they have ranked the items and why and then give them the expert's answers, which are:

ACTIVITIES

1 Two 100 pound oxygen tanks	you must breathe before you can do anything else
2 Five gallons of water	you must drink, you have got 200 miles to go, on the light and hot side of the moon – very thirsty work carrying your equipment
3 Stellar map of the moon's surface	this is your only means of getting about: even without food, with the map, water and oxygen you could reach the mother ship; you would be very hungry but you could do it
4 Food concentrate	200 miles is a long way on an empty stomach
5 Solar-powered receiver/transmitter	your best means of contact and guidance
6 50 foot of rope	for keeping together and climbing
7 First aid kit	it is going to get rough
8 Parachute silk	shelter from the sun's rays
9 Life raft	on which to drag all that heavy gear around
10 Signal flares	when you are nearer to home
11 Two pistols	sound doesn't carry as far as light
12 Dehydrated milk	not as good as the food concentrate
13 Heating unit	only useful if you were on the dark side of the moon
14 Magnetic compass	wouldn't work on the moon
15 Matches	no oxygen, so wouldn't strike on the moon

This is the expert's view, but it is still open to question: every time I think about it I rank it differently.

SNOWBOUND

Again split into small groups — create the scenario and provide props so that members get into the feel of things; then let them know that they are in a mess. It is late November and you are walking and camping with three friends in the Cairngorms.

You are now at the end of the fourth very long day and you are thoroughly cheesed off. You have been stuck in your tent for 24 hours since it started to snow. Visibility is now very limited and it is getting colder all the time and snowing harder than ever. You are worried because your tent is beginning to disappear under the snow and one of your group is beginning to show signs of hypothermia. They are shivering, their skin is pale and cold, and they are acting strangely, not making any sense and becoming drowsy. The nearest help is about 15 miles away through the snow. Visibility is now very poor with a near gale force north-easterly wind creating blizzard conditions.

The resultant snow drifts make the conditions treacherous, especially as the snow is covering uneven ground, boulders, gullies and scree.

You are faced with a series of choices. Regrettably, however, you did not inform anybody of your route before setting out and with poor visibility no-one will find your tent. In the foreseeable future the weather shows no signs of improving and your friend with hypothermia is getting delirious, and shivering constantly. Your only chance of survival depends on getting help. You have twenty articles available to help you, of which you must take ten and leave ten behind. The choice of what you take and leave will be crucial to the survival of all four of you. You must also decide who should go and stay and of course what first aid measures you should take for your friend with hypothermia. The twenty items are:

compass	torch
map	120 feet of rope
four sleeping bags	four Mars bars
three packets of soup	whistle
small first aid kit	watch
penknife	one ice axe
two bars of Kendal Mint Cake	primus stove
matches in waterproof box	large polythene bag
book, *The Advanced Scout Guide*	two flares
two rucksacks	one pair of binoculars

Now leave your group to sort this little mess out. The best response in this situation is clearly that two should go and two should stay. Two have a better chance of finding help provided they don't get separated and clearly someone has to stay and look after the hypothermia victim.

The first aid treatment until help arrives is:

1 Remove any wet clothing and replace it with dry;

2 Try to insulate from underneath the casualty by placing two sleeping bags under them and putting them in another one. You lose much heat from your contact points with the ground;

3 Lie beside the casualty inside the sleeping bag if you will fit so that you can pass on your body heat;

4 If the hypothermia victim is conscious, give hot drinks if possible.

Now the ten items you should take are listed below in order of priority:

1 **Compass** essential for accurate route finding. Work out a good route in the tent with your map and head off on your first bearing.

2 **Map** in case you get lost again and also because you've marked the position of the tent on it, haven't you!

3 **Rucksacks** essential for carrying your other gear, leaving your hands free. Can also be used for sitting on and you could try and get in it if you're stuck overnight (not as daft as it sounds as I know from bitter experience).

4 **Polythene bag** for an easy shelter if weather necessitates it and you get stuck overnight. Could also be used as a sledge.

5 **Mars bars** a good psychological boost, they are reassuring and boost your energy levels quickly.

6 **Watch** useful for judging distance covered and preventing distortion of time.

7 **Rope** for keeping in contact in poor visibility, river crossing, climbs, drops and so on.

8 **Torch** useful for signalling and a psychological aid if you are stuck overnight.

9 **Ice axe** for testing depth of snow.

10 **Whistle** signalling device.

The position of the tent is known, so as long as the other two stay put, they will be rescued. The soup can be heated on the primus stove to provide a warm drink for the hypothermia victim. The Kendal Mint Cake will give energy. The sleeping bags will keep you warm. The flares can be used if rescuers are heard. You can amuse yourself reading *The Advanced Scout Guide* so that you won't make the same mistakes again.

You can vary this simulation by changing the degree of misfortune and the scenario: for example, a broken leg in the middle of Dartmoor one very foggy February night.

DESERT RATS

It is midsummer in the middle of the Gobi Desert. You have just crash-landed your light aircraft because you didn't put enough fuel in it and now all that remains is the burnt-out frame and a few charred bits of wood and rubber. You know that you are 65 miles off course and that the nearest village is 70 miles away due south over the barren desert. The air temperature is 44°C (112°F) and the surface of the sand is roughly 54°C (130°F). There are three of you and you are all wearing shorts, light shoes and shirts. Between you you have got three biros, a packet of cigarettes, £3.20 in coins, and £26.00 in notes, but there are no taxis in sight. You have sixteen items available from the wreckage which you must put in order of importance to help you reach the village:

torch	pen knife
aerial map of area	large plastic raincoat
compass	bandage and gauze
pistol	red and white parachute
1000 salt tablets	one litre of water
book about edible cacti	two bottles of vodka
three overcoats	cosmetic mirror
three pairs of sunglasses	Max Bygraves' greatest hits album

I am not going to prioritize these: you can argue it out amongst yourselves.

Groupwork with elderly people, indeed with anybody, should not always be deadly serious. The most lighthearted games can be therapeutic. It just depends on what you want from that exercise. Getting people to interact can be your goal — how you get there is immaterial as long as it is either interesting or amusing. It need not even be that really; you could bore the pants off people and they would interact with each other: "This is boring — shall we go and have a cup of tea?"; hey presto, they are interacting.

However you run the risk of half of them falling asleep, so I would suggest that you err on the interesting side.

One of the things I have milked dry for many a lighthearted session is the field of horoscopes and fortune telling.

HOROSCOPES

Go around the group asking what sign people are and whether they take any notice of the stars. Do they believe in them? Now, dealing with each star sign in turn, read out the characteristics of that star sign personality and ask the group members if they have those characteristics.

Aquarius: the water bearer: from 20 January to 18 February

Like wandering and variety (itchy feet), easily upset and slow to forgive. Like rules but not losing.

Pisces: the fish: from 19 February to 20 March

Prosper best away from their birthplace. Make good wives and mothers. Vigilant and virtuous.

Aries: the ram: from 21 March to 20 April

A good sign to be born under, so they say. Their children will be dutiful but they themselves will be short-tempered.

Taurus: the bull: from 21 April to 20 May

Industrious and patient even when under much pressure. Men are bold, adventurous and fond of governing, but hard to please.

Gemini: the twins: from 21 May to 20 June

A good sign for women, who will be lucky in marriage. This sign denotes the qualities of punctuality, honesty, respect and the propensity towards having many children.

Cancer: the crab: from 21 June to 20 July

If you are born under this sign and have a fair complexion you will be exalted in life. Brunettes, however, will be prone to whims, jealousies and to being over particular.

Leo: the lion: from 21 July to 21 August

A good sign if you are born poor but not if you are born rich, because it denotes a change of fortune in your life. The poor usually marry into money.

Virgo: the virgin: from 22 August to 22 September

Men are brave, generous and honest. Women are likable and prosperous, but prone to flattery. They marry early (usually Leos) and have good children.

Libra: the scales: from 23 September to 22 October

A smooth, trouble-free, life. Faithful in love, smooth in transactions. Few children but healthy ones.

Scorpio: the scorpion: from 23 October to 22 November

Men are destined for a long, active and useful life. They are intelligent, prosperous and careful, make good husbands and parents. Women have the knack of becoming acquainted with those who are successful.

Sagittarius: the archer: from 23 November to 20 December

Both sexes are prone to an amorous disposition and love variety. Often don't marry and if they do it is late in life. After youth's follies they become steady and prudent and gather good friends about them.

Capricorn: the goat: from 21 December to 19 January

Hard workers but others tend to reap the benefit of their labours. Marrying another Capricorn portends a hard fate. After many obstructions and mishaps your later life will be more prosperous.

Obviously the next thing to do is to read out the day's forecast from the papers and check out the likelihood of the predictions.

FORTUNE TELLING

We move on now to fortune telling, but first I must give my source. It is a book I bought in an antique shop a few years ago called *Royal Fortune Teller*. It has no date of publication. I only hope it is past copyright date.

THE CARDS

This has to be done individually but the rest of the group will be interested to see what the cards foretell for others and will be dying to have their cards read. You can have one of the group read yours at the end.

Begin by shuffling the cards: this always gives the impression that you know what you are doing. Shuffle the cards three times. Ask the participant to choose four cards at random from the deck. It is these cards which are significant:

The 10 of hearts is a sign of marriage or prosperity, 10 of diamonds a journey. The ace of diamonds signifies a ring, the ace of hearts means something to do with your dwelling, ace of clubs a letter. Beware of the ace of spades — it foretells grieving or quarrelling. Presumably the 10 of hearts with the ace of spaces means a quarrelsome wife. The 3 of hearts foretells a salute, 3 of spades tears; 10 of spades sickness, 9 of spades a disappointment or trouble. It is your misfortune if you get the 10 of hearts, ace of spaces and 9 of spades. The 9 of clubs foretells joviality and much revelling, 9 of hearts feasting; 10 of clubs travel by water; 5 of hearts a present, 5 of clubs a bundle . . . bundle of what — fun, trouble . . .? The 6 of spades foretells a child; 7 of spades a removal; 3 of clubs fighting; 8 of clubs confusion, 8 of spades a road; 4 of clubs a strange bed; 9 of diamonds, business; 5 of diamonds a settlement, 5 of spades a surprise; a red 8 new clothes; 3 of diamonds speaking with a friend; 4 of spades sickness; 7 of clubs prison; 2 of spades a false friend; 4 of hearts marriage.

Several diamonds together is a sign of money; several hearts love; several clubs drink and bad company; and several spades vexation and trouble.

This venerable source of information then goes on to say that this method of using the cards is 'both innocent and will afford you amusement, while that common, destructive, and most pernicious habit of gaming, would otherwise tend to promote and complete the ruin of both your soul and body' . . . to say nothing of your wallet.

DOMINOES

Place all the dominoes face down and shuffle them — only once this time. Ask the participant to pick three. Then reveal their destiny thus:

6,6   money comes your way

6,5   fun

6,4 legal troubles

6,3 a bus journey

6,2 new clothes

6,1 a friend needs your help

6,0 beware of scandal

5,5 a new house

5,4 a fortunate speculation

5,3 a visit from someone in authority

5,2 a party

5,1 love

5,0 a funeral

4,4 drink

4,3 a false charm

4,2 beware swindlers

4,1 debts will be called in

4,0 a letter

3,3 a sudden wedding

3,2 your luck is down

3,1 you will make a discovery

3,0 a child

2,2 a jealousy

2,1 a promise

2,0 no significance

1,1 something to your advantage

1,0 no significance

0,0 the worst domino — it means trouble will come soon . . .

On that happy note we leave the realms of prophecy.

Section C

WORD GAMES & QUIZZES

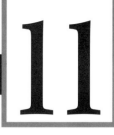
Word games cover a multitude of sins and can be used in many different ways. The emphasis here, as elsewhere, should be on fun. Without humour, they can become profoundly boring. It is also important, as it is with quizzes, to match the activity you choose, and the way you do it, to the intellectual level at which your client group is functioning. Some of the following categories are very useful with dementia sufferers, especially when backed up by large, clear pictures. However, to use them with a group whose intellectual function is intact would be both insulting and downright boring. The opposite is also true: do not use concepts which are beyond the grasp of your dementia sufferers as this will be perplexing and will serve only to enhance feelings of failure and worthlessness. I indicate those which I feel are of value in dementia groups (I stress again the use of pictorial clues), but in the final analysis only you will know your group.

SIMILES

Some of these are easy as pie, others as hard as nails. Many of the similes listed below can be used to stimulate discussion; for example, why is mustard said to be keen, and why are brushes daft?

As bald as a coot	As brave as a lion
As happy as a lark	As busy as a bee
As fat as a pig	As meek as a lamb
As mad as a hatter (or March hare)	As stubborn as a mule
As patient as Job	As quick as a flash
As wise as an owl	As thick as a brick (or thieves)
As strong as an ox	As sober as a judge

As daft as a brush	As quiet as a mouse
As pleased as Punch	As proud as a peacock
As slippery as an eel	As bold as brass
As slow as a snail	As cold as ice
As happy as a sandboy	As old as the hills
As safe as houses	As pretty as a picture
As thin as a rake	As drunk as a lord
As fit as a fiddle	As straight as an arrow
As dry as a bone	As sharp as a razor
As hard as nails	As clean as a whistle
As keen as mustard	As sound as a bell
As bold as brass	As flat as a pancake
As high as a kite	As steady as a rock
As right as rain	As cool as a cucumber
As hot as a vindaloo	As light as a feather
As good as gold	As clear as a bell
As fresh as a daisy	As bright as a button

Colours form a useful subsection of their own:

As white as snow	As black as coal (as the ace of spades)
As red as a ruby (or beetroot)	As green as grass
As blue as the sky	As brown as a berry

OPPOSITES

Some of the more obvious ones here can be of value with dementia groups and can be used in assessing degrees of cognitive deficit.

Summer	— Winter	First	— Last	
Dry	— Wet	Yes	— No	
Morning	— Afternoon (or Evening)	Stop	— Go	
In	— Out	Near	— Far	
Up	— Down	Rich	— Poor	
King	— Queen	Win	— Lose	
Back	— Front	Weak	— Strong	
Hot	— Cold	Open	— Closed	
Solid	— Liquid	Sad	— Happy	
Men	— Women	Top	— Bottom	
For	— Against	Thick	— Thin	
On	— Off	Young	— Old	
Over	— Under	Day	— Night	
Big	— Little	Fast	— Slow	
True	— False	Right	— Wrong (or Left)	
New	— Old	High	— Low	
Over	— Under			

The use of pictures here can be of obvious value for dementing people. You can discuss what the picture depicts before finding the matching picture.

RAMANAGS (ANAGRAMS TO YOU!)

You can make anagrams out of anything. In the category of towns etc adapt your local place names. Use group members' names to see if they can recognize themselves:

Towns/cities/states

Donlon	— London	Rapis	— Paris
More	— Rome	Diffcar	— Cardiff
Gagowls	— Glasgow	Rolifcaani	— California
Kooty	— Tokyo	Swocom	— Moscow
Collinn	— Lincoln	Bunild	— Dublin
Ghubriden	— Edinburgh		

Animals

Rede	— Deer	Worc	— Crow
Gerit	— Tiger	Grof	— Frog
Dersip	— Spider	Noli	— Lion
Act	— Cat	Woc	— Cow
Heros	— Horse	Heeps	— Sheep
Tar	— Rat	Yonmek	— Monkey

Countries

Genramy	— Germany	Danaca	— Canada
Lawes	— Wales	Icarema	— America
Danleng	— England	Sodnalct	— Scotland
Nicha	— China	Talyi	— Italy
Danleri	— Ireland	Canref	— France

Colours

Gerano	— Orange	Wolley	— Yellow	
Nereg	— Green	Klabc	— Black	
Hewit	— White	Leprup	— Purple	
Livers	— Silver	Lube	— Blue	
Der	— Red			

Plants

Lognaami	— Magnolia	Dewse	— Swede	
Koa	— Oak	Chinsap	— Spinach	
Trocar	— Carrot	Abbecag	— Cabbage	
Pilut	— Tulip	Amotot	— Tomato	
Tupane	— Peanut	Fafdilod	— Daffodil	
Prodsown	— Snowdrop	Cier	— Rice	

Obviously you could carry on for ever. The overenthusiastic amongst you will delight in making them as unrecognizable as blessiop.

GROUPS

A group of groups (collective nouns):

A shoal of herring	A suit of clothes
A troupe of dancers	A swarm of bees
A wisp of snipe	A pride of lions
A flock of birds or sheep	A gaggle of geese
A brood of chickens	A school of whales
A covey of grouse	A plague of locusts
A drove of cattle	A pack of wolves
A herd of cows	A litter of pups

A sheaf of arrows	A hand of bananas
A skein of wool	A wad of notes
A host of angels	A gang of thieves
A peal of bells	A nest of machine guns
A bale of cotton	A bunch of fives
A flight of steps	A fleet of ships
A diagnosis of doctors	A cluster of diamonds
A company of actors	

PAIRS

Parents	Offspring
Fox	Cub
Goat	Kid
Deer	Fawn
Frog	Tadpole
Sheep	Lamb
Cat	Kitten
Horse	Foal
Owl	Owlet
Eel	Elver
Lion	Cub
Goose	Gosling
Chicken	Chick
Swan	Cygnet
Elephant	Calf
Seal	Calf
Hare	Leveret

Partners: useful with dementia groups in conjunction with pictures

Bill and Ben	Jack and Jill
Gilbert and Sullivan	Tarzan and Jane
Antony and Cleopatra	Robin Hood and Maid Marion
Popeye and Olive Oyle	Laurel and Hardy
Lennon and McCartney	Lone Ranger and Tonto
Morecambe and Wise	Adam and Eve
Jekyll and Hyde	Holmes and Watson
David and Goliath	Cain and Abel
Samson and Delilah	Luke and John
Bonnie and Clyde	Tom and Jerry
Bootsie and Snudge	Flanagan and Allen
Romeo and Juliet	Rodgers and Hammerstein
Ginger Rogers and Fred Astaire	Abbot and Costello
Bing Crosby and Bob Hope	Little and Large
Napoleon and Josephine	Frankie and Johnny
Richard Burton and Elizabeth Taylor	Matthew and Mark

SOUNDS AND ORIGINATORS

Bird	Sings or whistles	Dove or pigeon	Coos
Owl	Hoots	Turkey	Gobbles
Duck	Quacks	Bee	Hums or buzzes
Cat	Purrs or miaows	Cow	Moos or lows
Dog	Barks	Donkey	Brays (hee-haws)
Frog	Croaks	Bear	Growls

Horse	Neighs or whinnies	Cock	Crows
Pig	Grunts or snorts	Lion	Roars
Crow	Caws	Wolf	Howls

EVERYDAY OBJECTS

This is a useful one for people who are dementing. Using common household items and simple concepts cut out pictures from magazines and stick them on card. The idea then is to get your clients to match them up. This can give you a useful guide to the severity of dementia and keep an eye open for any deterioration.

Toothbrush	Toothpaste	Bat	Ball
Knife	Fork	Cup	Saucer
Bread	Butter	Table	Chair
Fish	Chips	King	Queen
Soldier	Gun	Hat	Coat
Dustpan	Brush	Dog	Bone
Flowers	Vase	Needle	Cotton
Wellies	Umbrella	Bacon	Eggs
Socks	Shoes	Bird	Nest
Paper	Pen	Eyes	Glasses
Child	Toy		

Obviously we could go on and on. You can buy sets of photo cards depicting pairs but they tend to be quite small. A good supply of magazines should keep you busy for a while, though.

HOMES

Horse	Stable
Lion	Den or lair
Squirrel	Drey
Fox	Earth or lair
Monk	Monastery
Nun	Convent
Abbot	Abbey
Priest	Rectory
Otter	Holt
Spider	Web
Soldier	Barracks
Eskimo	Igloo
Gipsy	Caravan
Red Indian	Wigwam
Chicken	Coop
Dog	Kennel
Pig	Sty
Rabbit	Burrow or warren
Badger	Sett or earth
Bee	Hive
Beaver	Lodge
Cow	Byre

MR / MRS

MR	MRS
Stallion	Mare
Peacock	Peahen
Landlord	Landlady
Buck	Doe (rabbit)
Boar	Sow (pig)
Bull	Cow
Billy goat	Nanny goat
Boy Scout	Girl Guide
Dog	Bitch
Ram	Ewe
Stag	Hind
Colt	Filly
Gander	Goose
Cob	Pen (swan)
Sir	Madam
Lad	Lass
Master	Mistress
Lord	Lady
Abbot	Abbess
Sultan	Sultana
Duke	Duchess
Marquis	Marchioness
Brave	Squaw
Gentleman	Lady
Czar	Czarina
King	Queen

There are many things you can do with a good proverb or colloquialism. The obvious quiz routine is to get the group to finish off the proverb that you began. You can then move on to discuss what on earth it means and whether or not you think it holds true.

PROVERBS

Many proverbs contradict each other, or suggest that what one indicates may not be the best policy. It is useful to explore these and discuss situations in which each might be true. Examples of contradictory proverbs are:

1 Too many cooks spoil the broth — *yet* — Many hands make light work;

2 Look before you leap — *yet* — he who hesitates is lost;

3 Out of sight, out of mind — *but* — Absence makes the heart grow fonder;

4 Clothes maketh the man — *whilst* — Beauty is only skin-deep;

5 What's good for the goose is good for the gander — *whilst* — One man's meat is another man's poison;

6 The pen is mightier than the sword — *but* — Sticks and stones may break my bones, but words will never harm me;

7 Better to be safe than sorry — *but again* — He who hesitates is lost.

You will find many more yourself, but the emphasis in the group should be on stimulating discussion about whether or not the proverbs are true and what exactly they mean. Groups of dementia sufferers may enjoy merely finishing off and recognizing the proverb; so here are a few:

Better to be safe than sorry;

It never rains, but it pours;

A change is as good as a rest;

Money is the root of all evil;

One rotten apple can spoil the barrel;

You can't teach your grandmother to suck eggs;

It is no good bolting the stable door after the horse has bolted;

You can take a horse to water, but you can't make him drink;

He who hesitates is lost;

Half a loaf is better than no bread;

No use keeping a dog and barking yourself;

The grass is always greener on the other side;

A watched pot never boils;

It's no use crying over spilt milk;

A leopard can't change his spots;

People who live in glass houses shouldn't walk around in the nude;

Many hands make light work;

Make hay whilst the sun shines;

It is better to travel hopefully than to arrive;

Forewarned is forearmed;

Do not tell tales out of school;

Blood is thicker than water;

When the cat's away the mice will play;

Where there's a will there's a way;

Little boys should be seen and not heard;

You never miss the water until the well runs dry;

Look after the pennies and the pounds will look after themselves;

Unity is strength;

All work and no play makes Jack a dull boy;

Look before you leap;

Two heads are better than one;

A bird in the hand is worth two in the bush;

More haste, less speed;

Truth will out;

A friend in need is a friend indeed;

Too many cooks spoil the broth;

The early bird catches the worm;

Necessity is the mother of invention;

A rolling stone gathers no moss;

Still waters run deep;

New brooms sweep clean;

A stitch in time saves nine;

Spare the rod and spoil the child;

Absence makes the heart grow fonder;

Shoemakers' wives are worst shod;

No news is good news;

Actions speak louder than words;

No smoke without fire;

Set a thief to catch a thief;

Out of sight out of mind;

All that glitters is not gold;

Empty vessels make most noise;

All's fair in love and war;

Once bitten, twice shy;

He who pays the piper calls the tune;

One good turn deserves another;

Pride goes before a fall;

Out of the frying pan into the fire;

Better late than never;

Let sleeping dogs lie;

Birds of a feather flock together;

Charity begins at home;

It's an ill wind that blows nobody any good;

Cut your coat according to your cloth;

Discretion is the better part of valour;

In for a penny in for a pound;

Don't put all your eggs in one basket;

Don't count your chickens before they are hatched;

Flattery will get you nowhere;

Enough is as good as a feast;

Hunger is the best sauce;

Great oaks from little acorns grow;

Every cloud has a silver lining;

Great minds think alike;

Every dog has its day;

Forbidden fruit tastes sweetest;

Fine words butter no parsnips;

First come first served.

COLLOQUIALISMS

These are the nucleus of a good discussion group with regard to what they actually mean and many group members will know of local variants:

A fly in the ointment;

A red letter day;

Tell it to the marines;

Swing the lead;

A far cry;

Come a cropper;

As the crow flies;

Live from hand to mouth;

A white elephant;

Chewing the fat;

With flying colours;

Haul over the coals;

Turn over a new leaf;

Send to Coventry;

Pull your leg;

Let the cat out of the bag;

Be put through the mill;

Turn the tables;

Put the cart before the horse;

Rub up the wrong way;

Slinging mud;

Smell a rat;

Nip in the bud;

Mind your p's and q's;

Send packing;

The apple of your eye;

Hit the nail on the head;

A wet blanket;

Blow your own trumpet;

Get carried away;

Hit below the belt;

A chip off the old block;

Play the game;

Under a cloud;

Put your foot in it;

Down in the mouth;

Sit on the fence;

All ears;

Beside yourself;

Face the music;

At a loose end;

Silver-tongued;

Make both ends meet;

Lion-hearted;

Keep your powder dry;

At loggerheads;

Draw the line;

An old salt;

A rough diamond;

Have a bee in your bonnet;

Lead a dog's life;

Lead up the garden path;

Sweep the board;

Cold shoulder;

Turncoat;

Make no bones about it;

Show a clean pair of heels;

Throw in the towel;

Burning the candle
at both ends;

Have your heart
in your mouth;

Throw your cap at;

Bury the hatchet;

A feather in your cap;

Make a clean breast of it.

Quizzes are an integral part of any day centre because the scope of subject matter can be tailored to suit any client group. They can be great fun whilst at the same time being of immense value in assessing cognitive deficits.

You do not just have to ask questions. You can have many different formats for a quiz. The best way of making any quiz more enjoyable is by using as many pictures and props as possible.

There are many good quiz books on the market, covering a whole range of abilities and which can be easily adapted for particular client groups. The following are some variations on the straightforward 'what's the answer?' quiz.

Geography is left for later, where it occupies a chapter to itself.

CRISS CROSS QUIZ

A hugely successful group. This is noughts and crosses. Draw a large grid on the blackboard and divide the group into two teams. They have to answer a question correctly to get either a O or a X and then decide where to put it. Vary the questions by using all of the quiz ideas in this book, for instance, smells, pictures and abbreviations.

PICTURES

This section deals with the use of pictures and outlines three useful categories. The list of categories is endless. The three mentioned here are useful in reminiscence groups and by far your best resource is a large supply of magazines.

FAMOUS FACES

Make a scrapbook of famous faces or stick magazine photographs onto pieces of card so that they can be passed around. You can buy sets of famous faces cards ready made or over a period of time you can build up your own stock of glossy colour or black and white pictures cut out from magazines. It is useful to have a short biography of the person in question as well. You can then get the group to identify either the portrait or the history. *Empire Magazine* has recently published a series of supplements on film stars which are large and clear — excellent for our purposes. There are also many books full of large pictures available, often obtainable from 'bargain' bookshops. For reminiscence purposes I would also suggest you go to a few antique or book fairs where for only a few pounds you can get old cinema annuals. One useful and enjoyable variation is to cut from magazines small pictures of famous people and number them, stick them all onto a sheet of A4 size paper and photocopy one for each group member. They write the identities on the sheet and as a group go through them afterwards. This can be done for a huge number of different categories and can be an enjoyable regular weekly feature.

PLACES

Sources of pictures here are many; Sunday supplements and magazines are very good, as are tourist information centres. Old calendars and postcards are also excellent. However, the best source of worldwide photos of different places, free, is your nearest travel agent. I have had many a strange look directed at me as I have filled a carrier bag with holiday brochures from all over the world and staggered out of the shop under the weight. But it is well worth it — you can make excellent collages of different countries given this wonderful resource.

WILDLIFE

Again magazines and Sunday supplements are a good source. Harangue any nature lovers and bird watchers for their old magazines. Although you usually do not stand a chance of seeing any, travel brochures often depict native wildlife. This is another area in which there are many cheap glossy books on which it is worth spending a few pounds.

GRID QUIZ

Draw a bingo card on the blackboard, as in Figure 3, numbering the squares 1 to 20. Divide your group into two teams and allow one question per team alternately. Pick out numbers from 1 to 20 at random. A correct answer wins that square. If the first team gets it wrong offer that number to the opponents. If both get it wrong put the number back in the bag. A line or all four corners wins the game.

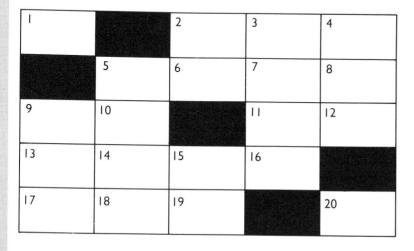

Figure 3 *Bingo*

CROSSWORDS

You either hate these or cannot leave them alone. Personally I cannot sleep if there is one clue left unsolved.

For our purposes it is useful to have a large blackboard, about a yard square, with the grid painted on it. Thirteen squares down and across is the usual pattern. This leaves you to just blank out the appropriate squares and put in the numbers. Occupational and industrial therapy departments of hospitals will usually oblige you by making one of these boards. Having a board this size ensures that everyone can follow the progress of the crossword without having to continually pass a paper around. It is also good because you can use chalk and rub out your errors!

The good thing about crosswords, and I repeat myself without regret, is that they are non-threatening. They are easy for people to join in with and it is up to you how much pressure you put on people. You can leave them to sit and watch or you can occasionally say, "What do you think, Jim?". The emphasis is on fun and doing something together.

ALPHABET LISTS

An easy one this, but often a very frustrating one. Write the alphabet on a blackboard, allowing enough space next to each letter for a word to be written. Then choose a category, such as names, towns, plants, animals, food. Then go down the alphabet, giving one thing for each letter. Q, U, V, X, Y and Z are often difficult. Again this is good fun, not greatly demanding and allows the shy ones opportunity to join in.

One excellent A–Z category to use is song titles, especially if you have got a pianist available (if not you will just have to hum the tune). This provides a good excuse for a sing-along. When you are stuck, the pianist or 'hummer' gives the tune for that letter and the group has to guess it. Then, when you have had the tune, you might just as well sing a few verses.

LETTER BOX

Draw a large grid on a blackboard five deep and six across. Ask the group for four categories, such as names, towns, vegetables and games, and write them in the four down spaces on the left. Then ask for five letters from the alphabet. Put these in the five spaces across the top. The group then has to fill in the blanks, as in Figure 4.

Letters / Categories	B	G	O	V	Y
TOWN	Birmingham	Greenwich	Olney	Ventnor	York
BIRD	Buzzard	Greenfinch	Oriole	Vulture	Yellow hammer
FLOWER	Begonia	Geranium	Ox-eye Daisy	Violet	Yarrow
GIRL'S NAME	Belinda	Gertrude	Olive	Veronica	?

Figure 4 *Letter Box*

I SPY

Choose a letter, then ask the group to shout out anything they can see beginning with that letter. (Ex-members of the I Spy Club should declare themselves before the game.)

WHAT'S IN A NAME

Take one of the group member's names, for instance Danny Walsh, and from that make as many different words as possible, for example, dawn, wash, lawn, day, wand, hand and so on.

ABBREVIATIONS

This is a good game because it can be used as a team quiz or brainstorm, and you can use it as a full activity or just to pass the odd twenty minutes. Using the list below (or alternatives that are suitable for your clients) just write the abbreviations on the blackboard and ask the group to supply the answer:

AA	Automobile Association
AB	Able bodied seaman
AD	Anno Domini
am	Ante meridiem (morning)
BA	Bachelor of Arts
BBC	British Broadcasting Corporation
BC	Before Christ
BR	British Rail
BSc	Bachelor of Science
CBI	Confederation of British Industry
CID	Criminal Investigation Department
Dr	Doctor
DSO	Distinguished Service Order
EEC	European Economic Community
eg.	For example (exempli gratia to you!)
ER	Elizabeth's Regina
etc	Et cetera

FA	Football Association		PS	Post scriptum
GB	Great Britain		PT	Physical training
GMT	Greenwich Mean Time		PTO	Please turn over
GPO	General Post Office		QC	Queen's Counsel
HMS	Her Majesty's Ship		RAC	Royal Automobile Club
HP	Hire purchase		RAF	Royal Air Force
hp	Horse power		RC	Roman Catholic
HRH	His or Her Royal Highness		RIP	Rest in peace
ie	That is		RN	Royal Navy
IOU	I owe you		RSPB	Royal Society for the Protection of Birds
JP	Justice of the Peace		RSPCA	Royal Society for the Prevention of Cruelty to Animals
lbw	Leg before wicket		RSVP	Répondez s'il vous plaît — reply if you please
Ltd	Limited			
MA	Master of Arts		SA	Salvation Army
MC	Master of Ceremonies		SAS	Special Air Service
MCC	Marylebone Cricket Club		TA	Territorial Army
MD	Doctor of Medicine		TUC	Trades Union Congress
MP	Member of Parliament or Military Police		UK	United Kingdom
NB	Notez bien — Note well		UN	United Nations
No.	Number		USA	United States of America
OAP	Old Age Pensioner		v	Versus
OBE	Order of the British Empire		VAT	Value Added Tax
OHMS	On Her Majesty's Service		VC	Victoria Cross
OK	All correct		YMCA	Young Men's Christian Association
PC	Police constable			
PM	Prime Minister			
pm	Post meridiem (afternoon)			
PO	Post Office			

This list is by no means exhaustive; one thinks, for example, of all the different trade unions, each known commonly by its abbreviation, for example, NALGO, NUPE, COHSE.

A NUMBER QUIZ

1	How many wonders of the world?	7
2	How many gospels?	4
3	How many commandments?	10
4	How many deadly sins?	7
5	Life begins at . . .	40
6	Unlucky for some	13
7	How many ages of man?	7
8	How many dimensions?	3
9	How many senses?	5
10	How many apostles?	12
11	How many blind mice?	3
12	How many green bottles?	10
13	How many players in a football team?	11
14	How many players in rugby union?	15
15	How many players in a rugby league team?	13
16	A stitch in time saves . . .	9
17	The naughty . . .	90s
18	A baker's dozen	13
19	How many dalmations?	101
20	How many does it take to tango?	2
21	Sweet little	16
22	Days in the year	365
23	Kelly's eye number	1
24	Downing Street number	10

What you need here are large simple maps and plenty of pictures.

You will be amazed at where people have been, many having travelled widely in the war. One word of warning, though: some of the group will not have travelled. One of our chaps always got asked where he had been and he always used to say, "We were too poor to have holidays." He said it very forlornly and he said he felt sad when everyone else was relating their travels. He was too poor, he came from the slums in the East End of London and he deserved not to be reminded of it. This having been said, travel is a useful subject matter for stimulating discussion and for quizzes. One excellent source of visual aids and pictures for quizzes and collage is your local travel agent.

Even those who have not travelled can take part in the quizzes and there are many different ways of doing a geography quiz or discussion; the following are just a few.

MAPS

With a large map of the world or Europe you ask people to name the major seas, continents, countries, capitals, rivers, landmarks, for instance the Taj Mahal, and get them to locate them on the map. You can enlarge maps using a photocopier but it is better to buy a world map and trace it onto a large sheet of paper so that everybody can see it. You can then mark things on as people identify them.

PICTURES

Using your travel agent's brochures, cut out the best pictures and make sheets of collage representing various countries, cities, cultures and so on, the group guessing where it is as you do your collage and using it as a springboard for discussion. Would you like to live there? Has anybody been? What is the national currency, diet, wildlife, dress?

QUESTIONS

There are a million and three things you can ask about the world, but the obvious things are:

1 **The continents**
Europe, Asia, Africa, America, Australasia (sometimes called Oceania), Antarctica (often included as the sixth continent).

2 **The oceans**
The Atlantic (divided into north and south), Pacific, Indian, Arctic and Antarctic.

3 **The lakes**
The largest are the Caspian Sea (Asia), then Lake Superior (America), Victoria Nyamza (Africa) and the Aral Sea (Asia).

4 **Mountains**
The highest is Everest at 29,028 feet. Most of the others that come anywhere near this are in Tibet, Nepal or India in the Himalayas range, but other famous ones are Kilimanjaro in Tanzania, Africa at 19,340 feet, which ranks only number 43 in height; Mount Ararat, where the Ark landed in Turkey at 16,946 feet; Mont Blanc in France at 15,781 feet. In Britain, the highest, Ben Nevis, is a paltry 4,406 feet.

5 **Rivers**
The longest is said to be the Nile at 4,160 miles, second is the Amazon at 4,080 miles, third is the Yangtse in China at 3,964 miles, fourth is the Mississippi (Missouri) at 3,740 miles.

14

Other famous rivers are the Danube, no. 26 at 1,770 miles; no. 31 is the Ganges at 1,560 miles; no. 44 is the Rhine at 820 miles. Our own Thames is a mere 158 miles from the Houses of Parliament to its source.

6 Country sizes

The largest used to be the USSR at 22,402,000 square kilometres; second Canada at 9,976,147; third is China at 9,561,000; fourth the USA at 9,363,130; fifth is Brazil at 8,511,968 and sixth Australia at 7,682,300. The UK is only 244,104.

7 Populations

The largest population belongs to China, with 1,005,000,000; second comes India with 750,900,000; third was the USSR with 282,300,000; the UK has only 56,600,000.

CURRENCIES

Australia	— Dollar		Belgium	— Franc
Canada	— Dollar		China	— Yuan
Denmark	— Krone		Egypt	— Pound
France	— Franc		Germany	— Deutschmark
Greece	— Drachma		Holland	— Guilder
India	— Rupee		Italy	— Lira
Japan	— Yen		Mexico	— Peso
South Africa	— Rand		Spain	— Peseta
Russia	— Rouble			

MAP ONE

	Country		Capital
1	Eire	—	Dublin
2	Northern Ireland	—	Belfast
3	Scotland	—	Edinburgh
4	England	—	London
5	Wales	—	Cardiff
6	Portugal	—	Lisbon
7	Spain	—	Madrid
8	France	—	Paris
9	Belgium	—	Brussels
10	Luxembourg	—	Luxembourg
11	Holland	—	The Hague
12	Germany	—	Berlin
13	Denmark	—	Copenhagen
14	Switzerland	—	Zurich
15	Italy	—	Rome
16	Austria	—	Vienna
17	Czechoslovakia	—	Prague
18	Hungary	—	Budapest
19	Poland	—	Warsaw
20	Albania	—	Tirane
21	Greece	—	Athens
22	Romania	—	Bucharest
23	Bulgaria	—	Sofia
24	Turkey	—	Ankara
25	Crete	—	Iraklion

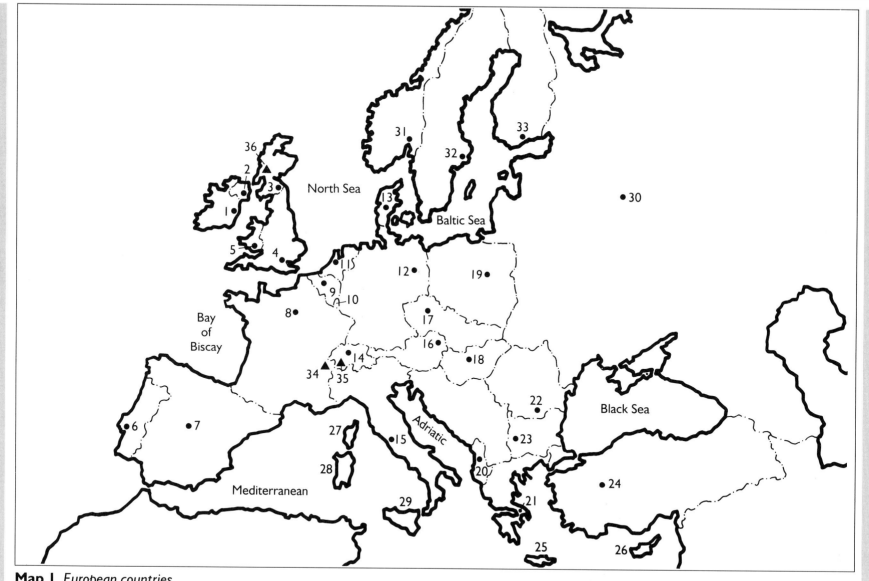

Map 1 *European countries*

26	Cyprus	—	Nicosia
27	Corsica	—	Ajaccio
28	Sardinia	—	Cagliari
29	Sicily	—	Palermo
30	Russia	—	Moscow
31	Norway	—	Oslo
32	Sweden	—	Stockholm
33	Finland	—	Helsinki

Mountains
34 Mont Blanc
35 Matterhorn
36 Ben Nevis

MAP TWO

1 British Isles	8 Russia
2 Europe	9 Australia
3 Canada	10 New Zealand
4 United States of America	11 Japan
5 South America	12 China
6 Africa	13 Mexico
7 India	

Capitals and other major cities

14 Buenos Aires	19 Cairo
15 Brasilia	20 Addis Ababa (Ethiopia)
16 Mexico City	21 Canberra
17 Washington DC	22 Sydney
18 Ottawa	23 Casablanca

24 Peking	29 Wellington
25 Tokyo	30 Moscow
26 Bombay	31 Singapore
27 Calcutta	32 Hong Kong
28 Delhi	

Mountains

33 Everest	35 Kilimanjaro
34 Mont Blanc	36 Ararat

Lakes

37 Caspian Sea	39 Victoria Nyanza
38 Lake Superior	40 Aral Sea

Rivers

41 Mississippi	44 Ganges
42 Amazon	45 Yangtse
43 Nile	

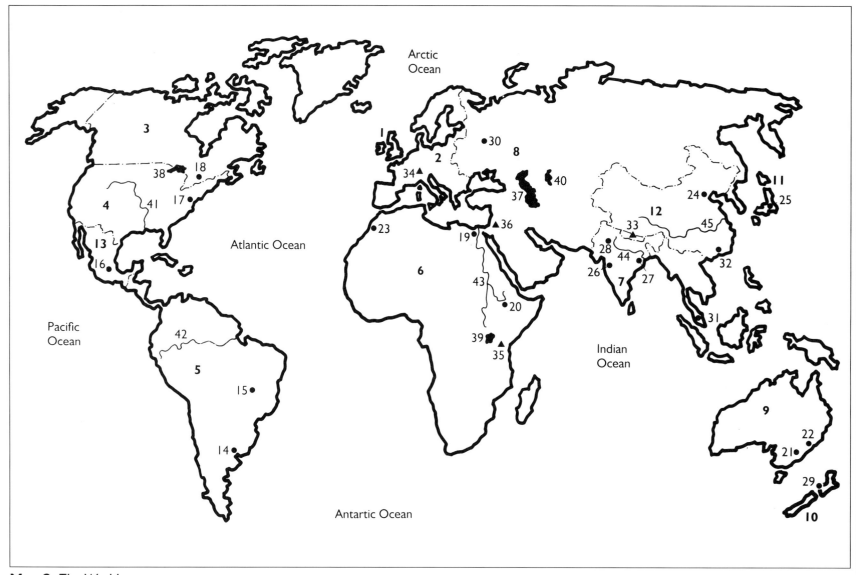

Map 2 *The World*

14

OUTLINES

This is an interesting variation whereby you present the outline of a country and ask the members to guess it. They can be easily traced or photocopied and enlarged. What I usually do is hold them upside down or sideways to make it just that bit more difficult.

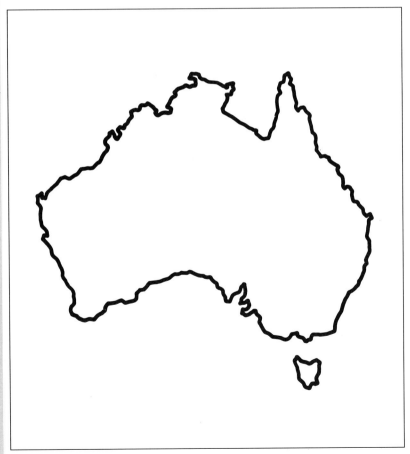

Australia

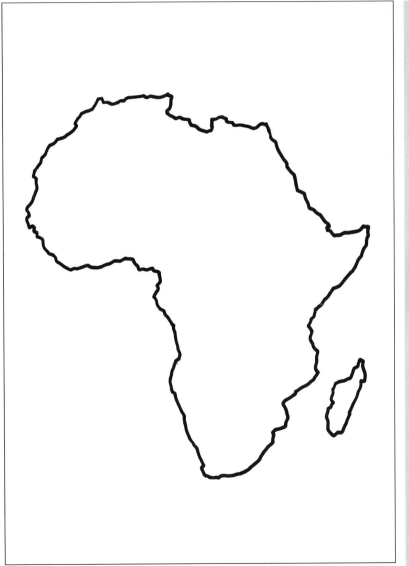

Africa

14

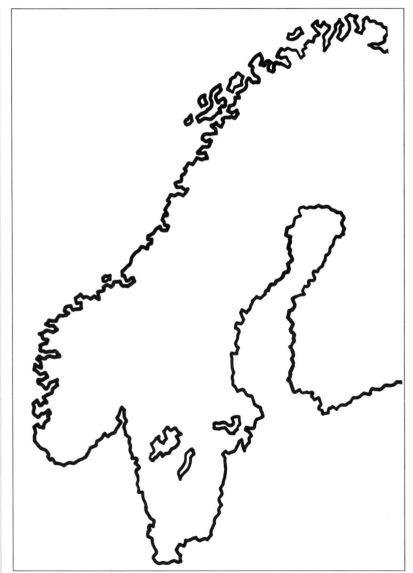

Scandinavia

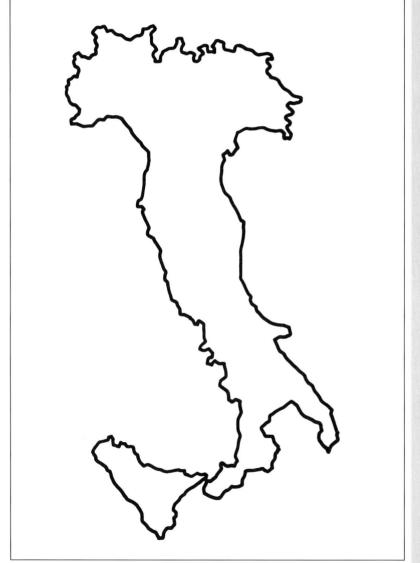

Italy and Sicily

14

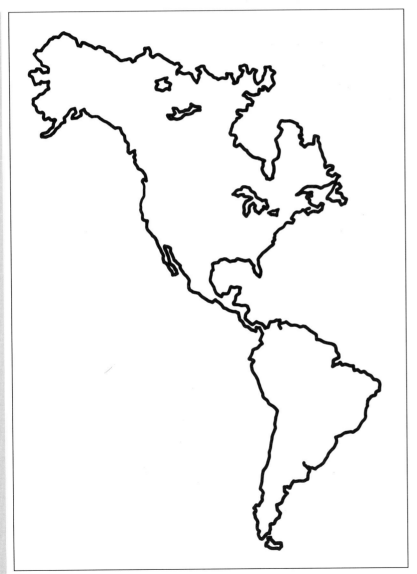

Canada, North and South America

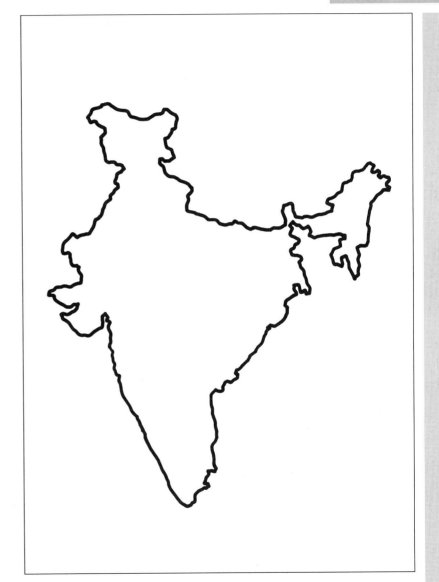

India

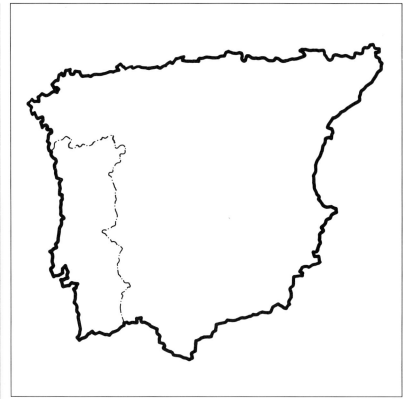

Spain and Portugal

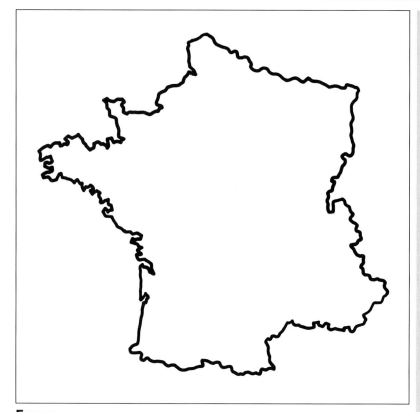

France

ACTIVITIES

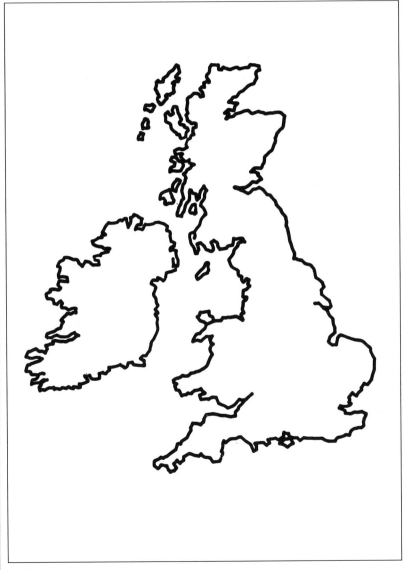

British Isles

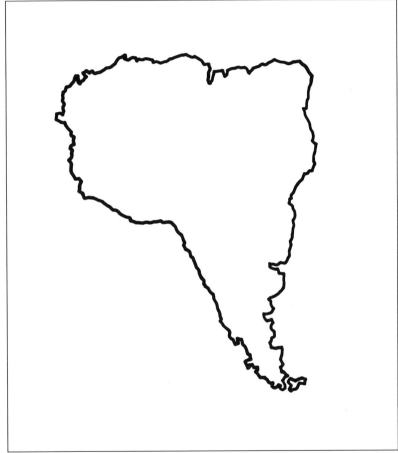

South America

OTHER VARIATIONS

Again using travel brochures, compile sets of pictures of the wildlife — both plant and animal — of various places and use these for a group or quiz questions. You can also use national costume, food and customs.

To look at an individual country can be a successful focus for a group as there are so many questions you can ask and ways you can think about it. Here are some ideas for the British Isles, but any country can be used by just substituting relevant examples. Use travel agents and tourist information centres for getting together a collection of large pictures representing the major landmarks and tourist attractions as well as building a local profile.

It is useful to have a large outline map painted on a blackboard so that you can mark the position of various places on it as they arise in discussions. You can also use it for quizzes by marking features on it. Then wipe it clean and you still have your outline left. With the British Isles it is amazing how difficult it is to draw it from memory and there is an interesting group here. Just ask each member to draw the British Isles — pin them up and compare with a map.

Themes you can use are: where I was born, where I have lived, where I went for my holidays.

The following maps show some of the major cities, rivers and other features, but again I emphasize the usefulness of pictures to back up any questions and discussion.

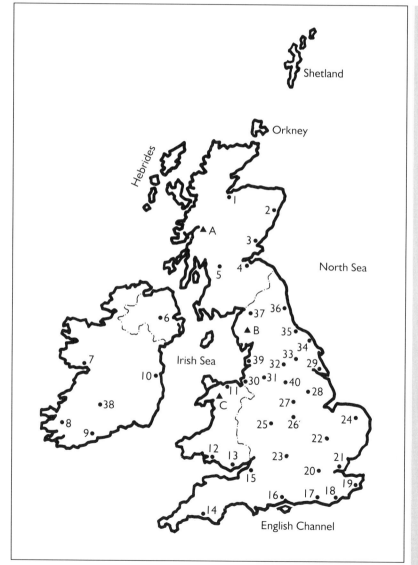

Map I

MAP 1

Mountains

A Ben Nevis
B Scafell Pike
C Snowdon

Cities and other places of interest

1	Inverness	21	Southend-on-Sea
2	Aberdeen	22	Cambridge
3	Dundee	23	Oxford
4	Edinburgh	24	Norwich
5	Glasgow	25	Birmingham
6	Belfast	26	Leicester
7	Galway	27	Nottingham
8	Killarney	28	Lincoln
9	Cork	29	Hull
10	Dublin	30	Liverpool
11	Llandudno	31	Manchester
12	Swansea	32	Leeds
13	Cardiff	33	York
14	Plymouth	34	Scarborough
15	Bristol	35	Middlesbrough
16	Southampton	36	Newcastle
17	Brighton	37	Carlisle
18	Hastings	38	Tipperary
19	Dover	39	Blackpool
20	London	40	Sheffield

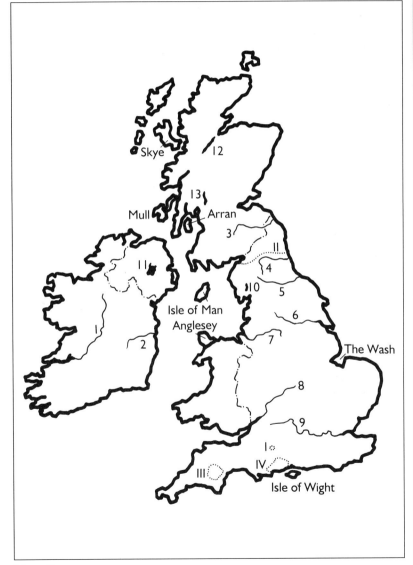

Map 2

MAP 2

Rivers

1	Shannon	6	Humber
2	Liffey	7	Mersey
3	Tweed	8	Severn
4	Tyne	9	Thames
5	Tees		

Lakes

10	Windermere	12	Loch Ness
11	Lough Neagh	13	Loch Lomond

Features

I	Stonehenge	III	Dartmoor
II	Hadrian's Wall	IV	New Forest

BRITAIN QUIZ

1	Where did William the Conqueror give one in the eye to Harold?	Hastings
2	Where could you be sent in silence and Lady Godiva rode naked through the streets?	Coventry
3	Where did the British fleet sail from to defeat the Armada, when Drake had finished playing bowls?	Plymouth
4	Which city is the home of steel?	Sheffield
5	Where would you not sell coal?	Newcastle
6	A lake with a monster	Loch Ness
7	Blue birds flew over its cliffs	Dover
8	Home of the Mersey beat and the Beatles	Liverpool
9	An illuminated northern seaside resort with a famous tower	Blackpool
10	Starting point of a famous march of the unemployed in the depression of the 1930s	Jarrow
11	Dick Whittington was its mayor	London
12	Where you could once run away to get married	Gretna Green
13	The granite city of Scotland	Aberdeen
14	Home of the 'bull ring', Cadbury's chocolate, Aston Villa, BSA and Spaghetti Junction	Birmingham
15	Home of the pavilion and famous for its 'belles'	Brighton
16	On the river Avon, with its Clifton suspension bridge, Temple Meads station and the birthplace of Concorde	Bristol
17	Its impressive castle, overlooking the Menai Straits, is where Prince Charles was invested	Caernarfon

18	On the river Cam, with a famous university, where you can row along the 'backs' and under the Bridge of Sighs	Cambridge
19	A cathedral city in Kent where St Thomas Becket was murdered and to which pilgrims progress	Canterbury
20	Capital of Wales and where the 'Arms Park' is the home of Welsh rugby	Cardiff
21	Where there are: Cowes you cannot milk Freshwater you cannot drink Newport that cannot be bottled Needles you cannot thread and where you can get a ticket to Ryde!	Isle of Wight
22	Here you will find Douglas, cats without tails and a three-legged man	Isle of Man
23	A Scottish town famous for its cake, and its two bridges over the river Tay	Dundee
24	Scotland's capital with its Royal Mile, arts festival, castle, Princes Street and Greyfriars Bobby	Edinburgh
25	Where the druids meet at the solstice — built of large stones in the Bronze Age	Stonehenge
26	Largest city in Scotland on the Clyde, renowned for its shipbuilding and the Gorbals	Glasgow
27	Home of 'United' — Busby's Babes and Coronation Street	Manchester
28	Capital of the fens, home of Colmans mustard and famous for its canaries	Norwich
29	Robin Hood hid in its Sherwood Forest but never went to its famous goose fair	Nottingham
30	Where the Thames is called Isis and the university likes to row	Oxford

31	Home of the potteries	Stoke
32	William Shakespeare's home and where you can find Anne Hathaway's cottage	Stratford-upon-Avon
33	Home of the Shambles and famous for its minster	York
34	In its fair city the girls are said to be so pretty — home of Guinness and Eire's capital	Dublin
35	It's a long way to there, so they say, to the sweetest girl I know	Tipperary

ACTIVITIES

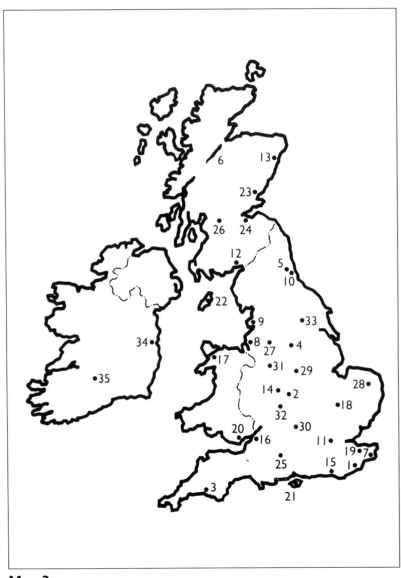

Map 3

MAP 3

Locations (can be used in conjunction with the Britain Quiz)

1	Hastings	19	Canterbury
2	Coventry	20	Cardiff
3	Plymouth	21	Isle of Wight
4	Sheffield	22	Isle of Man
5	Newcastle	23	Dundee
6	Loch Ness	24	Edinburgh
7	Dover	25	Stonehenge
8	Liverpool	26	Glasgow
9	Blackpool	27	Manchester
10	Jarrow	28	Norwich
11	London	29	Nottingham
12	Gretna Green	30	Oxford
13	Aberdeen	31	Stoke
14	Birmingham	32	Stratford-upon-Avon
15	Brighton	33	York
16	Bristol	34	Dublin
17	Caernarfon	35	Tipperary
18	Cambridge		

Section D

EXERCISE & RELAXATION

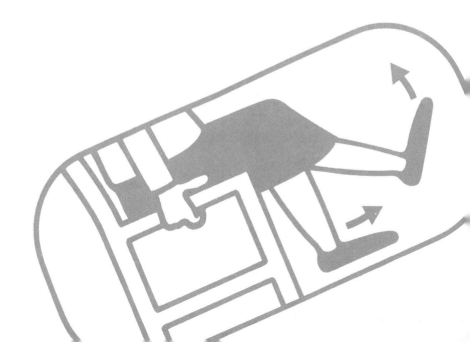

I do not want to dwell too long here. There is very little I can do but offer a few suggestions.

First of all, bowls. Bowls is very easy. Throw the little white ball and see how near you can get with the bigger balls. You can buy cheap sets of 'boules' and spend many a summer afternoon on the grass, or playing indoors — you can even do it from the comfort of your chair.

Another useful semi-energetic pursuit which can be played from the safety of your armchair is quoits. Croquet is relatively sedentary and with a little imaginative use of wheelchairs can also be played seated. Indoor hockey is good. Sitting in a circle, everyone brandishing a hockey stick and thrashing wildly at anything that moves within eyeshot is good fun. A set of twelve plastic sticks can be purchased from professional therapy catalogues, or you can get your nearest hospital therapy department to make you some wooden ones.

Bean bags are a resource that is greatly underrated. One enjoyable and physiotherapeutically valuable exercise is merely having a floor target at which to aim. Placing a bin in the middle of a painted drawsheet is a good idea.

On a more sedentary note, a large balloon (a metre or yard across) which can be bounced around the room is a good way of getting the arms going. Foam or other soft balls, of football size, are also good for tossing around a circle, shouting the name of the person to whom you are aiming it.

Hoops thrown over cones, like a large version of quoits, is also good fun.

Skittles is a good game too, for which there is no need to stand up. Skittles can be bought cheaply from toy stores and are great fun. But the last word must go to the humble bean bag. Mark lines on the floor about 3, $3\frac{1}{2}$, 4 and $4\frac{1}{2}$ metres (10, 11, 12 and 13

feet) away. The aim is to slide your bean bag along the floor into the 5, 10, 25 or 50 point areas.

We have only touched upon a few of the many games which are traditionally played either outside or from a standing position. The key to success in many areas of life is adaptability and this is particularly so here. In much the same way that having fun is not contraindicated by dementia, being active is not exclusively the preserve of those who can get up and walk. By being adaptable you can use whatever is at hand to widen the experience of your clients, and any exercise gained in the process is secondary to this goal.

Moving on to the more traditional indoor games, there is always going to be a time and a place for such games as bingo and dominoes. But they should not be relied upon and their use should be limited. Too often they rely on individuals concentrating on their state of play and not on people actively interacting with each other. By the same token we do not want to force interaction upon people all the time and we must remember that fun is a priority. So some ideas:

Cards	Dominoes	Draughts
Chess	Shove halfpenny	Scrabble
Solitaire	Tiddlywinks	I spy
Hangman	Connect 4	Othello

BOARD GAMES

There are some excellent board games on the market these days, for example Monopoly and Cluedo; Trivial Pursuit, although expensive, is worth its weight in gold and is a good standby when you are stuck, especially as a quiz source. Pictionary is another good one demanding a little abstract thought. There are also some good geography and general knowledge quizzes. Brit-Quiz is a good one — a race around Britain answering questions about

British geography, history and culture. You can get a good noughts and crosses made of small wooden pieces, which is ideal for our client group. However a browse around a good toy shop should supply you with many more ideas.

BINGO

For many bingo is a part of their culture and heritage and not just a game. Apart from the normal game you can have a useful group brainstorming the various bingo calls. An alternative way of playing is with two packs of cards — the dealer shuffles both and deals one pack equally among the players. He then calls out the cards from the other pack. The first to have all his cards called wins.

The bingo calls:

1 Kelly's eye
2 One little duck or buckle my shoe
3 On its own, up a tree, or sit on my knee
4 On its own, close the door, or knock on the door
5 On its own, or snakes alive
6 On its own, or pick up sticks
7 On its own, or go to heaven
8 On its own, shut the gate, or one fat lady
9 On its own, doctor's orders, or on a cloud
10 Downing Street
11 Legs eleven
12 One dozen
13 Unlucky for some
16 Sweet little sixteen
20 Blind 20

21 Key to to the door
22 All the twos, or two little ducks
26 Two and six — half a crown
30 Blind 30
33 All the threes
40 Blind 40
44 All the fours droopy drawers
50 Bull's eye, or blind 50
55 All the fives
59 The Brighton line
60 Blind 60
65 Time to retire
66 All the sixes clickety click
70 Blind 70
76 Seven and six — was she worth it?
77 All the sevens, or Sunset Strip
79 A glass of wine
80 Blind 80
88 All the eights, or two fat ladies
90 Top of the shop.

It is good fun to keep people on their toes, and to make sure no one is falling asleep throw in a few trick ones like:

All the eights	—	fifty-seven
On its own	—	blind thirty-four
Legs	—	forty-three
Three and seven	—	twenty-five

Exercise takes many shapes and forms, not all of them good for you. If at all possible get a physiotherapist to design routines customized to the capabilities of your clients.

Music, as in relaxation, can be a great help to liven up an exercise session and also make it feel more of a special activity.

With elderly people, and anyone else, exercises are designed to keep the muscles in trim and the joints flexible. Never do anything that could cause discomfort and pain.

In much the same way as you can tape relaxation exercises, you can photocopy a few pages of exercises so that people can do them at home if they wish.

The following exercises can all be done, with a little adaptation, from a chair. Another useful tip is to draw the diagrams on large sheets of paper so that folk understand your instructions.

1 Sitting on a chair, raise and lower the right leg six times. Repeat with the left leg. This will strengthen the muscles of the calves and thighs.

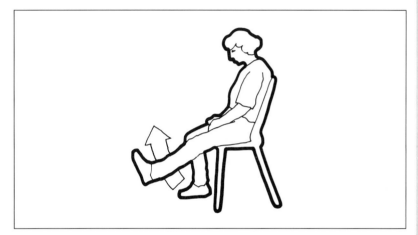

2 Lift your right knee up to your chest and hold it there with your arms. Do this three times and repeat with your left knee. This will strengthen your back and thighs.

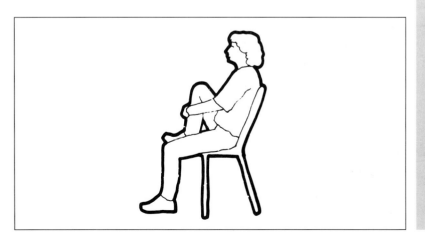

3 Point the toes of the right foot down and raise them six times. Repeat with the left foot.

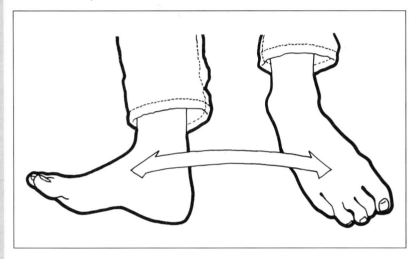

4 Turn the right foot inwards and then outwards six times. Repeat with the left foot.

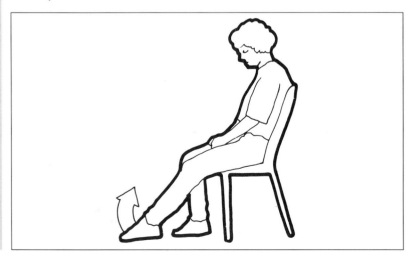

5 Move the right foot in a circular motion six times. Repeat with the left foot.

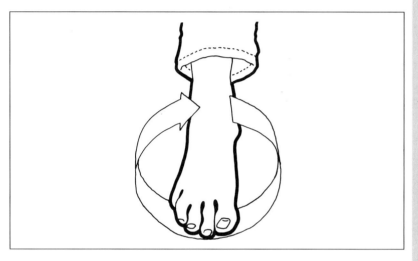

6 Bend and straighten the toes of the right foot six times. Repeat with the left foot.

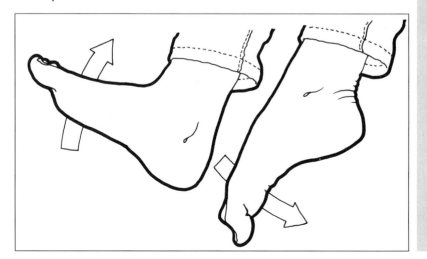

7 Swing your whole right leg in a circular motion three times in a clockwise direction, then three times in an anticlockwise direction. Repeat with your left leg.

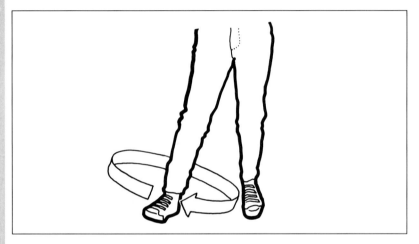

8 With the palms of your hands facing you, stretch your fingers wide, then press them tight together. Do this six times.

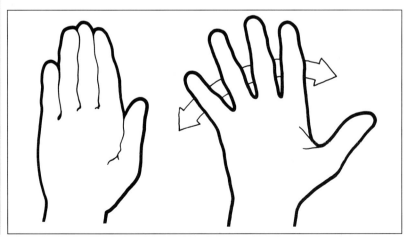

9 Touch each finger with your thumb individually on each hand. Repeat six times.

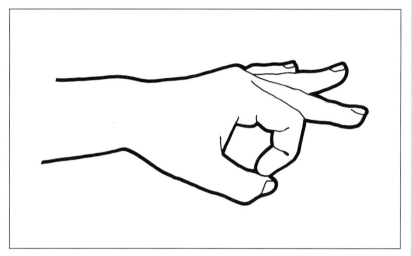

10 Make a fist with both hands. Squeeze them as tight as you can, then fling your fingers outwards.

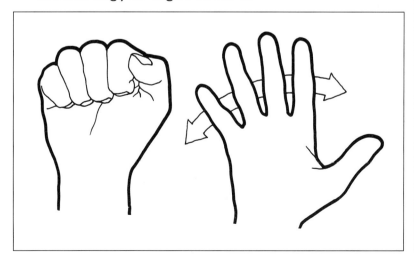

11 Bend your right elbow up to your shoulder. Bend and straighten six times. Repeat with your left elbow.

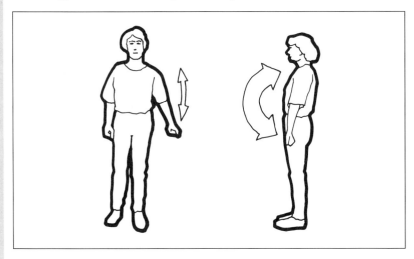

12 Arms outstretched in front of you. Twist both hands back and forth at the wrist. Repeat six times. Then palm up, palm down.

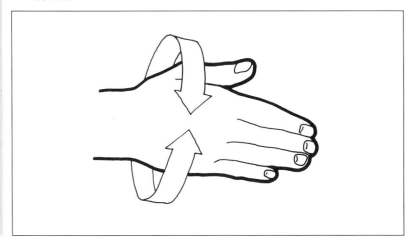

13 Holding your hands close to your chest like a kangaroo, allow the wrists to drop and fingers fall down. Then flick them up as far as they will go. Repeat six times.

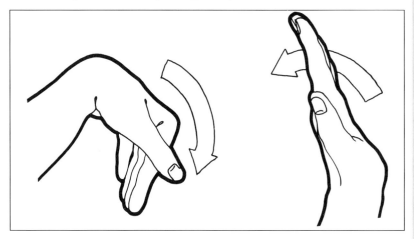

14 Bend your head as far forward as it will go and then as far back as it will go. Repeat six times.

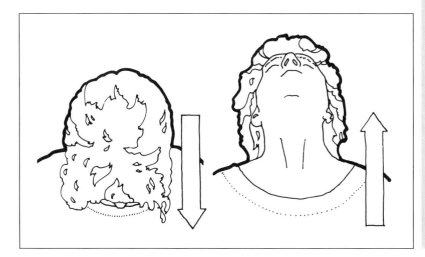

15 Bend your right ear towards your right shoulder then your left ear to your left shoulder. Repeat six times.

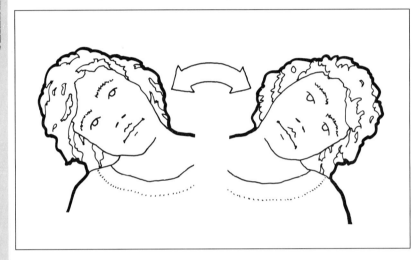

16 Turn the head to the left, then to the right slowly. Do this six times.

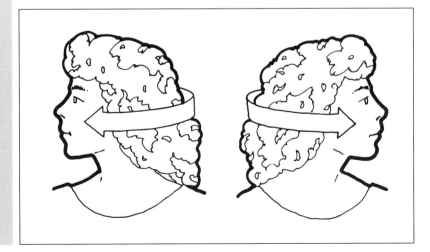

17 Shrug your shoulders up to your ears. Repeat six times.

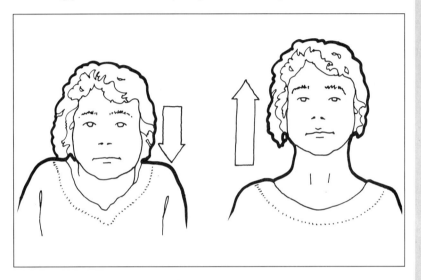

18 Stretch your arms down by your sides, then swing them up above your head. Repeat six times.

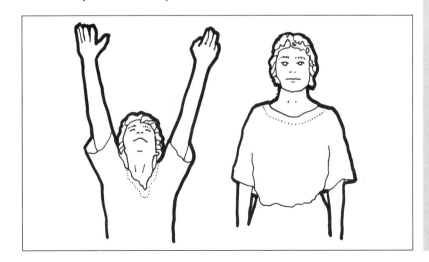

19 Pull in your stomach, then slowly let it all fall out. Repeat six times.

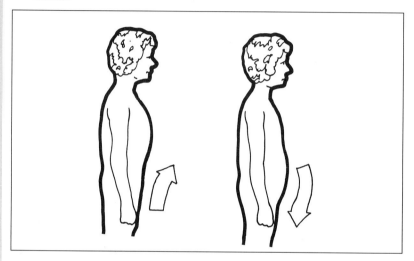

20 Screw up your face (eyes, nose and mouth) as tightly as you can. Then relax. Repeat six times.

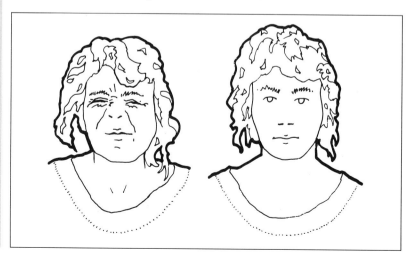

JUST STROLLING

Merely going out for a walk in the fresh air is a very enjoyable experience. It provides obvious exercise and can be combined with all manner of excuses. Collecting natural history objects (for example, feathers, flowers, leaves) for later use in collages or discussion is a favourite excuse to get people outside; but merely enjoying the fine weather is excuse enough. There are no groups described in this manual that cannot be carried on out of doors. Set the chairs out in a circle on the grass and have your interaction group there.

It is possible for everyone to go outside; Kirton chairs have castors fitted, beds have wheels.

Relaxation groups are excellent for elderly people. They not only provide an enjoyable group experience, they relax us and give us an awareness of our own bodies, and they are useful as exercise in their own right.

More therapeutically, relaxation exercises form an integral part of programmes attempting to diminish anxiety states. Teaching clients the techniques, so that they can assume a relaxed state at will, gives them an independence and control over their condition. Once they believe they can overcome small panics, that confidence helps them to master larger hurdles.

There are many different techniques and ideas about how relaxation should be done and you can buy tapes telling you what to do and taking you through the exercises. However I find it is best if you do all the talking yourself; tapes tend to sound robotic and impersonal, and doing it yourself gives you control over the pace of the session. You can always make someone a tape for home use quite cheaply and you can personalize it for them.

The formula I favour is where we create a scenario in the mind, for example lying on a soft sandy beach, with the seagulls wheeling overhead, the waves gently lapping at the beach, the warm sun caressing your face. Obviously you can vary this and it can become a fun part of the group, with the clients wondering what scenario you will dream up this week.

The basic technique aims to teach people how to relax and control their bodies by taking each muscle group in turn and working through a tensing and relaxing routine, whilst at the same time focusing on how they are breathing. Once learnt it can be readily used at home. Control over anxiety comes after you are familiar with the technique. Gradually you come to associate the relaxation learnt over muscles with calmness and freedom from anxiety.

Anxiety is a natural and useful force but it can get out of control and become destructive. Relaxation training helps your confidence grow. Fear of excessive anxiety and panic attacks diminishes as your confidence overrides the fear.

The technique then; first some ground rules:

1 It is not sacred — adapt it at will.
2 Privacy is essential in the beginning. Interruptions damage confidence and ruin the flow, any calmness achieved is immediately lost. Eventually you should be able to practise relaxation almost anywhere.
3 A darkened room is conducive to calmness (unless of course you are afraid of the dark).
4 Music is very much a matter of personal preference. I find that some classical pieces playing in the background help the atmosphere and make the 'group experience' more enjoyable. My preferences are:

Grieg	— Morning — Peer Gynt
Bach	— Air and Jesus Joy of Man's Desiring
Albinoni	— Adagio in G minor
Vaughan Williams	— Fantasia on Green Sleeves
Beethoven	— Pastoral Symphony

5 If possible have everyone lying on the floor, but if this is not possible due to frailty then sitting in comfortable armchairs is fine. Explain the nature and purpose of the session and then begin.

Now down to business.

1 Put the chosen music on at a low volume. Ask the participants to make themselves comfortable, eyes closed, arms by sides and legs uncrossed. Explain we are going to be focusing on all the major muscle groups, tensing them and relaxing them and concentrating on our breathing. What follows is more or less your script.

"Breathe softly and slowly and as you breathe in think of and feel the goodness of the air, savour it like a fine wine, then as you breathe out focus on the word 'relax' and feel the tension flowing out of your body with the expelled air.

2 "Carry on breathing softly and imagine a warm sunny day with clear blue skies. You are on a small secluded beach soaking up the warmth. Hear the seagulls crying above you as they glide effortlessly around in the sky. Listen to the gentle lapping of the waves as they ripple upon the beach. Feel the warmth and comfort of the soft sand beneath you and just focus on the feeling of softness and warmth. Let your body relax and go limp.

3 "We are going to begin with our feet and lower limbs and gradually work our way up our body. Point your toes forwards and straighten your legs. Make them stiff, hold it, then relax and allow them to flop. Focus on the tension flowing down your legs and out through your toes. Be aware of your legs and feet, where they are in contact with the floor. Feel the support beneath them. Feel your legs becoming heavier and sinking into the sand. Let the tension flow out of them, feel their weight, let your feet roll outwards and relax. Every time you breathe out feel the tension flow away.

4 "Now arch your back up and squeeze your buttocks, feel the pent up tension, then let them go, sink back into the

floor, dropping deeper into its softness. Feel the tension flow down out of you.

5 "Now make your stomach muscles rigid, as if someone has aimed a blow at your stomach, feel the tight knot and tension — then breathe out and relax the muscles. Feel the relief in your stomach. Feel the warmth of the sun on your chest, breathe out the tension and feel it flow away. Feel yourself sinking deeper into the soft sand.

6 "Feel now how immobile you are from stomach down to buttocks, thighs, calves and feet. Feel how limp and relaxed they are. Feel that tension draining out down your body through your toes every time you breathe out.

7 "Now take a deep breath and hold it, hunch up your shoulders, feel the tension in your chest and shoulders. Breathe out slowly and feel your body sinking, your shoulders relaxing back into the soft warm sand. Feel how peaceful you are.

8 "Let your arms flop down and feel them supported by the sand, feel them getting heavier and heavier. Clench your fists and stretch your arms out. Feel the tension in your arms, then breathe out and let them drop back onto the warm sand. Let them go and feel the tension flowing out through your fingertips down into the sand.

9 "Feel your body sinking down into the soft sand, hear the seagulls overhead and the waves lapping the beach. Feel the sun on your face making you glow with warmth. Then breathe in and tense your neck.

"Push your head back and screw your face up tight. Feel the tension and anger, then let go. Relax. Breathe out and let all that tension drain away. As you breathe out feel the back of your head and neck sink into the sand, feel your face becoming peaceful.

10 "Let this feeling of relaxation spread all over your body. You can feel the warm support of the sand. Your whole body feels heavy and limp and free from tension. Breathe slowly and steadily, feeling the warm glow of the sun on your face. Now listen to the music gently playing, feeling peaceful and relaxed."

11 This is the end of the script. Let the group lie relaxed listening to the music for a few minutes, then say . . .

12 "We are going to slowly come back from the beach." So tell them to slowly feel their feet, wiggle their toes, roll their legs gently from side to side; to arch their backs a little just as if they were waking up in the morning. "Give a yawn, then stretch yourselves and slowly open your eyes. Then in your own time get up and smile at everyone else."

13 When all the members have become alert allow them time to discuss how they felt. "How was it for you?" Discuss any difficulties experienced and dismiss them lightly as unfamiliarities with the technique. Reassure them that mastery will come with practice. It does not work for everybody, so do not expect that it will.

Section E

THE ARTS

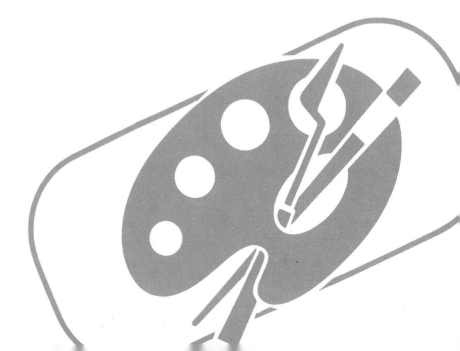

Poetry is strictly a matter of personal preference: you either love it or loathe it.

Poetry can be read and listened to for pure enjoyment, or it can be analysed and discussed.

There are many good poetry anthologies on the market and in the libraries. One good source of famous 'snatches' of poems is a dictionary of quotations. Group members may not wish to recite the poems and should not be made to; you will just have to cultivate your own style.

Here is a list of group favourites . . .

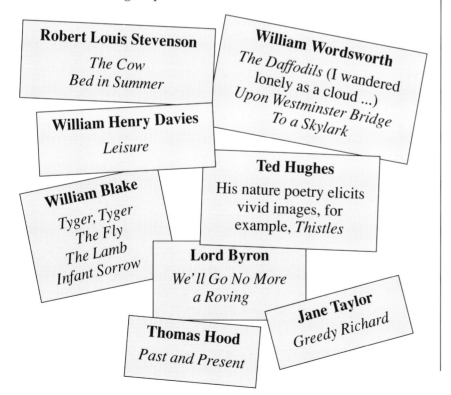

Robert Louis Stevenson
The Cow
Bed in Summer

William Wordsworth
The Daffodils (I wandered lonely as a cloud ...)
Upon Westminster Bridge
To a Skylark

William Henry Davies
Leisure

William Blake
Tyger, Tyger
The Fly
The Lamb
Infant Sorrow

Ted Hughes
His nature poetry elicits vivid images, for example, *Thistles*

Lord Byron
We'll Go No More a Roving

Jane Taylor
Greedy Richard

Thomas Hood
Past and Present

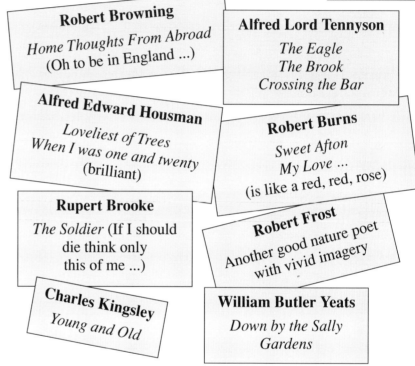

Robert Browning
Home Thoughts From Abroad (Oh to be in England ...)

Alfred Lord Tennyson
The Eagle
The Brook
Crossing the Bar

Alfred Edward Housman
Loveliest of Trees
When I was one and twenty (brilliant)

Robert Burns
Sweet Afton
My Love ... (is like a red, red, rose)

Rupert Brooke
The Soldier (If I should die think only this of me ...)

Robert Frost
Another good nature poet with vivid imagery

Charles Kingsley
Young and Old

William Butler Yeats
Down by the Sally Gardens

WRITING POETRY

This is worth a try if you have got a good group who enjoy the reading.

STORYTELLING

Again if you have a group which enjoys reading poetry it is worth trying a reading group. Books can be followed weekly, sharing the reading, or short stories can be read each week and discussed. Seasonal themes can be used: for example, Edgar Allan Poe at Hallowe'en. It is also worth bearing in mind that you can get books on tape, which relieves you and the members of the burden of reading.

ACTIVITIES

A good dictionary of quotations is what you need here. The breadth and range of quotations is enormous, from the profound to the ridiculous, the sad to the funny. Many are famous and many are obscure. Poets, politicians, the Bible, Shakespeare, they are all there.

You can use quotations for a quiz or just the sheer pleasure of listening to something 'well put', or for discussing the truth or otherwise of what is quoted. I always try to start and end the group with something amusing, for example:

'I feel no pain dear Mother, now
But oh I am so dry

Oh take me to a brewery
And leave me there to die'
Anon

Many of the quotations will elicit sayings from the group members themselves, for example, old rhymes from our school days. Others give general observations on life which can be discussed . . .

'What is this life, if full of care,
We have no time to stand and stare'
William Henry Davies

Or . . .

'There is so much good in the worst of us,
And so much bad in the best of us,
That it ill behaves any of us,
To talk about the rest of us'
Anon

Here are a few more to whet your appetite . . .

'Tis better to have loved and lost than never to have loved at all'
Alfred Lord Tennyson

'Hunger is the best sauce in the world'
Miguel De Cervantes

'Swans sing before they die
Twere no bad thing,
Did certain persons die before they sing'
Samuel Taylor Coleridge

'Tis better to die on your feet
Than to live on your knees'
Dolores Ibárruri

'I keep six honest serving men
(They taught me all I know)
Their names are what and why and when,
and how and where and who'
Rudyard Kipling

'The more I see of men,
The better I like dogs'
Mme. Roland

'Wagner has lovely moments,
But awful quarters of an hour'
Gioacchino Rossini

'Four be the things I'd been better without,
Love, curiosity, freckles and doubt'
Dorothy Parker

The following are more well known and can form the basis of a quiz.

1 Fasten your seat belts, it's going to be a bumpy night.
   Bette Davis

2 I want to be alone.
   Greta Garbo

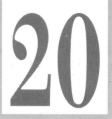

ACTIVITIES

3 If you want me just whistle,
You know how to whistle don't you.
Lauren Bacall

4 Here's looking at you kid.
Or
Play it again Sam.
Humphrey Bogart

5 Come up and see me sometime.
Mae West

6 Don't put your daughter on the stage Mrs Worthington.
Noel Coward

7 I came, I saw, I conquered.
Julius Caesar

8 We shall fight them on the beaches.
Or
Never in the field of human conflict was so much owed by so many to so few.
Winston Churchill

9 England expects that every man will do his duty.
Lord Nelson

10 Religion is the opium of the people.
Karl Marx

11 A week is a long time in politics.
Harold Wilson

12 Little things affect little minds.
Benjamin Disraeli

13 Let them eat cake.
Marie Antoinette

14 A horse, a horse, my kingdom for a horse.
Richard III by William Shakespeare

15 It is better to travel hopefully than to arrive.
Robert Louis Stevenson

16 I like work, it fascinates me, I could sit and look at it for hours.
Jerome K Jerome

17 Come into the garden Maud.
Alfred Lord Tennyson

18 I wandered lonely as a cloud.
William Wordsworth

19 I have nothing to declare but my genius.
Oscar Wilde

20 To be or not to be, that is the question.
Hamlet by William Shakespeare

21 No man is an island.
John Donne

22 Dr Livingstone I presume.
Sir Henry Morton Stanley

A useful aid here is the game 'Quotations', made by a company called Milton Bradley; it gives four packs of cards each with various quotes or quote related questions which can be used as a resource. Its 'Buzz words' pack can become a group game on its own. It gives you a word, for example, 'eggs', and what you have to do is come up with a proverb or saying which includes that word — so 'don't put all your eggs in one basket', or 'which comes first the chicken or the egg'.

Slides are a good way of making a group that little bit more of an event. We started out just using slides of flowers, wildlife and various places that staff had visited. It was such a success that it became a weekly event in the day hospital programme. Slides can be used in many ways, purely for enjoyment, quizzes, reminiscence, perception; the list is endless.

Do not exclude visually impaired people from the group. The subject matter and what conversation it stimulates is what is important here not the photograph *per se*. Have a staff member sit next to those with visual difficulties and ensure they vividly describe the slide content. This will elicit imagery in their minds and you can then get them to recall their own acquaintance with the subject matter. Here are some ideas for slide groups:

1 The Past

You can get good slides for a reminiscence session from organisations such as Help the Aged. In the UK Help the Aged produce a series covering *Childhood* (1920s), *Youth, The Great War, Living Through the 1930s* and *The Second World War*.

British Gas also produce a good set of slides on early gas appliances and other items, such as street lights, the gas works. You can get hold of these from Health Education centres, hospital and public libraries as well as buying them direct. Alternatively get a friendly photographer, or the local photographic society, to take slides of famous faces from the past using magazines (don't infringe copyright) and so on, and local land marks or any other subject.

2 Staff Slides

Your own and group members' own slides are a good source. If you have got a member of staff who is into natural history and photography you have cracked it. Wildlife, flowers, fungi, berries and so on, are all good material. More obviously slides of places people have visited can be used. Sessions we have found to be stimulating apart from those already mentioned are Scotland, Wales, Ireland, Europe, America, the coast, London, historic houses, castles, churches, children and animals. It is also useful to focus on the seasons.

3 Unusual Angles

You know the kind of thing — a close up of the underneath of a light bulb. You can make your own or ask a local photographic society to do it for you. It is also worth approaching your local art college or sixth form, as they may be able to do it as a project. You can use unusual angles of a:

light bulb	paint brush
toothbrush	box of matches
£10 note	cauliflower
plug	cheese grater
bunch of keys	feather
beer bottle	tap
book	apple
pen and pencil	tin opener
cigarettes	milk bottle

4 Local Landmarks

This speaks for itself. Again either take your own or get a local society or college to do some for you.

ACTIVITIES

5 Art

You can get slides of famous and not so famous paintings from art galleries, and the relative merits of each piece of work can be discussed.

6 Photographic Societies

This is art for art's sake. Ask the local photographic society to come and give a slide show of their members' work. This can be repeated at regular intervals. More importantly get them to do you a series of slides on various themes.

7 Animals

Good slides of animals can be bought from zoos and this is usually good fun.

8 Famous Faces

Again you can make your own here if you have got a decent camera. Just take slides of good magazine photos (take care over copyright). Alternatively use your local photographic society again.

VIDEOS

These are another way of varying the sessions. You can now get videos of the decades, for instance what happened in the 1940s, sport, politics, entertainment and so on. These are obviously a great source of stimulation for comments and observations. You can also video relevant television programmes on numerous themes. One good way of using videos is to get someone to video clips from famous films as they are shown on television. You will end up with a brilliant reminiscence and quiz resource.

FILMS

Finally a word about home movies. These are good because usually they are of family life and local events. Encouraging a client who has a good collection to show their films is a huge ego boost and provides a sense of importance and self-worth.

TRIPS

Usually on trips staff and clients take colour prints, but it is worth changing to slides which can then be wheeled out every now and again for a nostalgic film show.

There are many ways in which you can have a group based upon music and in which you can vary the degree of participation as is pertinent to your group members.

APPRECIATION

This is music for music's sake; just pure and simple listening for enjoyment. The enjoyment of music is often a faculty retained when others have been lost. It is undemanding and can bring to mind many memories. It creates a mental imagery and many thoughts and feelings can be stimulated by one piece of music.

CONCERTS

This is enjoyment again but of 'live' as opposed to recorded music. Either arrange in-house concerts or organise trips. Local choral societies can be used or school bands and so on.

QUIZZES

There are several types of musical quiz; some are outlined below, together with some questions you could use.

FIRST LINERS

Give the first line of a song and the group has to guess the title. Bonuses can be awarded for, say, singing the chorus. Here are a few first lines . . .

Underneath the lantern by the barrack gate.
Lilli Marlene

Should auld acquaintance be forgot.
Auld Lang Syne

In Dublin's fair city.
Cockles and Mussels

Come, come, come and make eyes at me.
Down at the Old Bull and Bush

And did those feet in ancient times.
Jerusalem

By yon bonnie banks and yon bonnie braes.
Loch Lomond

There's an old mill by the stream.
Nellie Dean

Where has thou been since I saw thee.
Ilkley Moor (Baht'at)

Oh we ain't got a barrel of money.
Side by Side

Once a jolly swagman camped by a billabong.
Waltzing Matilda

Private Perks is a funny little codger.
Pack up your Troubles

While the moon her watch is keeping.
All Through the Night

'Twas on a Monday morning.
Charlie is my Darling

Fierce the beacon light is flaming.
Men of Harlech

Alas my love you do me wrong.
Greensleeves

Oh give me a home, where the buffalo roam.
Home on the Range

It was late last night when the squire came home.
Gypsy Davey

Down away where the nights are gay.
Jamaica Farewell

Sur la point d'Avignon
Frere Jacques

COLOURFUL SONGS
What is the missing colour?

Ten . . . bottles

. . . roses, for a . . . lady

. . ., . . ., grass of home

Rudolph the . . . nosed reindeer

. . . Moon

. . . cliffs of Dover

. . . Christmas

. . . sails in the sunset

. . . rose of Texas

Bye, bye . . . bird

That old . . . magic

. . . Ridge mountains

Little . . . jug

Little . . . bull

. . . Sleeves

The . . . river valley

SONG PLACES

In . . . fair city

It's a long way to . . .

I belong to . . .

Tulips from . . .

Rose of . . .

Yellow rose of . . .

I left my heart in . . .

Maybe it's because I'm a . . .

White cliffs of . . .

Slow boat to . . .

. . . here I come

. . . races

My old . . . home

The man who broke the bank at . . .

On . . . moor baht'at

She's a lassie from . . .

Joshua fought the battle of . . .

The lass of . . . hill

The . . . poacher

Men of . . .

. . . farewell

COMPOSERS

1812	Tchaikovsky
Four Seasons	Vivaldi
Peer Gynt	Grieg
Blue Danube	Strauss
Carmen	Bizet
Pastoral Symphony	Beethoven
Karelia Suite	Sibelius
Water Music	Handel

William Tell Overture	Rossini
Marriage of Figaro	Mozart
Swan Lake	Tchaikovsky
The Planets	Holst
The Messiah	Handel
Bolero	Ravel
Enigma Variations	Elgar
Pictures at an Exhibition	Mussorgsky
Ride of the Valkyries	Wagner
Scheherezade	Rimsky Korsakov
Jesu, Joy of Man's Desire	Bach
Air on a G string	Bach
Hard Day's Night	Lennon and McCartney
Rhapsody in Blue	George Gershwin
Fantasia on Green Sleeves	Ralph Vaughan Williams
King of the Road	Roger Miller
Bridge over Troubled Water	Simon and Garfunkel
Blue Suede Shoes	Carl Perkins
West Side Story	Bernstein
Goodnight Irene	Huddie Ledbetter (Leadbelly)
Mr Tambourine Man	Bob Dylan

NAME THAT TUNE

This is exactly what it says. Guess the song. You can use tapes, and records, but it is good if you can procure the services of a piano player. Quiz, reminiscence, call it what you want, it is good fun. You can buy tapes of snatches of songs but eventually these wear very thin. Far better that you sit by the record player and act as disc jockey.

INSTRUMENTS

For this you require the services of a music college or school. Ask them to produce for you a tape of the sound of different musical instruments. Alternatively you can buy records or tapes of musical sounds, for example, 'The Young Person's Guide to the Orchestra'. Obviously the thing to do is have a quiz and discuss the various sounds.

SINGALONG

This, without a doubt, is one of the most enjoyable and best received things you can do. Consumer opinion dictates that this should be a regular event, though often the sound of staff wailing away out of time and out of tune may indicate otherwise. There are several ways to approach this. Obviously the best is to have a piano player; alternatively distribute musical instruments liberally amongst the participants and just start singing and banging away. Get the words printed from large print songbooks so nobody has any excuses for mumbling. One way to make it more of an event is to invite people from other areas in for that session and spend time beforehand baking and preparing teas.

TEA DANCE

Taking the singalong idea a little further, organize monthly tea dances. Try and get a band in or just use tapes, serve tea, sandwiches and cakes and have lots of dancing.

JUKE BOX JURY

This is based on the famous television show of that name. Simply play a selection of different tunes covering the various musical spheres and go around afterwards discussing the various merits or otherwise of the tunes. On a "would you buy it?" basis, declare them either a hit or a miss!

You can turn almost anything into a therapeutic activity. Art can be therapeutic, that cannot be denied, but it is not necessarily easy to analyse. In certain circumstances art can be used as a diagnostic tool — indicating gloom, for example, by weak, small, dull pictures, and rampant psychosis by Van-Gogh-cum-Dali-type creations. How we decide whether someone is rampantly psychotic or a genius, however, is tricky.

Suffice it to say that art can indicate much that is of value in getting to know something about the artist. This is not what we are concerned with primarily, though we will touch on this later.

What we are concerned with mainly is art as fun, creation and meaningful activity. Like many groups, the task in hand is secondary to the interaction it fosters, for example, the fun of doing something together and the mutual praise for each other's efforts. This is far more important than the relative merits of the work itself and such interaction helps build self-esteem and confidence. Having produced something seen as worthwhile by others our pride is boosted and we feel useful.

Art as part of reality orientation (see chapter 27) is useful. You can make huge collages three metres (10 feet) or so long and all admire it afterwards. Replace it weekly, cutting out the best bits.

In between, depending on the theme, we may have been reminded what time of year it is. It is in fact the middle of winter, it is snowing, very cold and there is a lot of ice about, the wind is howling, small birds are dying in their thousands, there is every chance of a power cut, nobody has got any candles and the buses are on strike. Cheerless! But we all join in, get to know each other better and 'art' makes it fun.

It is important also that the group leader does not frustrate, insult, or ridicule the client by trying to achieve a level of skill way beyond their capabilities or far below them. As in all groupwork, aim your tasks at particular ability levels with care.

Collages, I believe, are a wonderful experience for dementia sufferers in particular. They are hugely and widely applicable — you can make a collage out of almost anything as long as somehow you can stick it onto a piece of paper.

Your imagination is your only limit. The basis of collages are pictures cut from magazines and supplemented by other material; for example, a seasonal collage can be supplemented with feathers, nuts, conkers, grasses, ferns, flowers, leaves, fruits, twigs and so on.

All these things provide a bonus — feel them, smell them; you can even taste them if they are edible.

Anyhow, enough of collages, for a while at least. Where were we . . . ?

Right! Art for art's sake? Maybe not. We are not going to analyse the collage and say that the juxtaposition of the conker with the wood pigeon tail feather is deeply significant about how the group felt at that time, for such is fanciful speculation. But what we can do is give praise for ideas, pictures chosen and participation.

Occasionally, however, it can be useful to spend some time looking at paintings and discussing what we feel they say about the painter. This can provide useful feedback to the painter and be a good focus for discussion. It can also highlight the dangers of over interpreting and making assumptions about people. You can get a group around a table with some paper and paint and ask the group to paint how they feel today. After twenty minutes we can discuss the paintings one by one saying what we think the painting expresses — for example sadness, elation, insecurity, confidence. Such free interpretation can be a cause for discussion, and how we project ourselves on paper can lead us to reflect upon how we project ourselves in other ways.

But back to some more basic principles. Art and craft is not everyone's cup of tea. For some it is great, it provides a creative and enjoyable way of expressing themselves and an infinite variety of ways of doing it. However, asking someone to do some painting can often be an unwelcome suggestion. Do not expect overwhelming enthusiasm from everyone.

What follows is a list of various ideas which may or may not be appropriate for everybody or in every situation. It is down to you to decide what is pertinent and what is not. Just do not underestimate anybody or insult them by suggesting anything well below their capabilities. Remember there is nothing intrinsically therapeutic about art and craft if a person really does not want to do it. If they do, though, you can exercise their motor, perceptual, creative and cognitive skills, whilst at the same time remotivating and resocializing, but most of all enabling them to have fun.

COLLAGES

In order to make it more of an event you could try to run the group in a special room. It always helps if you go off the ward, or out of the lounge to another area for example. The order of the day then is giving the feeling of going somewhere special; start by having a cup of tea, introducing everyone to each other and, especially when working with elderly confused people, use a lot of touch in welcoming and talk away like you have just discovered your voice. It is worth emphasizing that active participation is not as important as staff often feel it ought to be. What is more important is that people feel they are involved in something of a social event.

So, the collage. Sit people in a circle and cut out your pictures from magazines. Make the circle as tight as possible so that everyone feels involved, but give yourself enough room for the three metres (10 feet) long collage in the middle.

With your large piece of paper on the floor have one of the staff in the middle sticking down the chosen pictures in places decided by the clients. Cover the whole thing with large pictures first, then put the smaller ones on top of them or covering any gaps — neatness is not an important consideration. What is important is the interaction between you and the clients as you are doing the collage. Go around the group individually helping them choose pictures, discussing what they are, why they like them — you will need at least two other helpers for this to keep everyone involved. More active members can do the cutting and glueing. Do not let it become a 'let's watch the staff make a collage' group. It needs and uses a lot of energy and moving between people in the face of possibly little apparent response. Non-respondents, by virtue of their more severe dementia, will pick up on a sense of being a part of a busy event. Holding up a picture and saying 'Can anybody tell me what this is?' will be very boring and will not involve those who cannot respond. Get on your knees and go around to everyone with the pictures as they are cut out. Tell them what the picture is and reiterate what is going on. "This is a nice picture, isn't it? It is a tulip, we'll stick it on the paper with the others, it's nice and bright isn't it?"

By doing this, even those who cannot or will not respond get a sense of activity, colour, movement, different environment, smells, sound, touch, exercise and general chaos. Though not actively participating, sitting as part of a group just watching the activity gives a sense of having done something and been some-where.

LIST OF COLLAGE THEMES

Spring	VE Day — 8 May
Chinese New Year	Burns Night — 25 January
Summer	Wildlife
Autumn	Gardening
Hallowe'en	Guy Fawkes
St Swithuns Day — 15 July	Poppy Day
Christmas Day	Ash Wednesday
Easter	Mothers' Day
St George's Day — 23 April	Fathers' Day
St Patrick's Day — 17 March	American Independence
St David's Day — 1 March	Day — 4 July
St Andrew's Day — 30 November	Bastille Day, France
Midsummer's Day	— 14 July
Plants	Countries
Pets	Places
People	Sport

Children	Winter
Fashion	Valentine's Day — 14 February
Transport	May Day
Town	

Jewish Festivals

Passover	Pentecost
New Year	Day of Attonement

Islamic Festivals

Ramadan	Id-al-fitr
Id al-adha	New Year

PHOTOCOPIES

Not all of us are blessed artistically and as soon as you say "We're going to do some art and craft" you invariably hear someone say "Oh, I'm no good, I can't draw to save my life!" One good way to get around this is by photocopying pictures for people to paint or colour. There are some excellent line drawings of various flower designs and many other subjects in books of tapestry and embroidery designs. This eradicates the fear of failure and those who cannot draw are usually pleased with their results. You can photocopy anything that takes your fancy as long as you do not infringe copyright. You can use art books and have people redesign the Mona Lisa or Constable's work. Landscapes from calendars are another good source.

SPLODGE PAINTING

This is a personal favourite. It is failure free and anyone can do it. Its beauty lies in the fact that people think they are creating a mess until the final moment. All you do is take a piece of paper and you get people to splash paint all over it, experimenting with different colours. Having created your mess, simply fold the paper in half and press it all over with your palms, then unfold it and you have a multicoloured symmetrical pattern. These nearly always look superb. Needless to say this is ideal for a confused elderly person. They can manage it easily, you can help them splash the paint if necessary and they are delighted with the results. You can ask people what the result reminds them of. For particularly vivid images use bold printing ink — using this method on pieces of card is quick and the results can be used to make greeting cards and so on.

STRINGFOLDS

This is pretty much a version of splodge painting and again, produces good failure free results and is ideal for elderly confused people. Gather various bits of string, cotton, wool and so on, soak them in paint and lay them on your piece of paper. Now fold the piece of paper in half and, pressing down on the paper, pull the string out from between the folded paper. Your result is a colourful and unusual symmetrical pattern.

POTATO PRINTING

We all know this from our school days and it is a good introduction to the principles of printing. Chop your potatoes in half (you can experiment with different vegetables) and carve your design into the flat surface. Mix a fairly thick solution of paint in a saucer or plate and dip your potato in and print away. If you want to be more refined about it place some thick tissue over your plate of paint. This will soak up the paint (make the paint a bit thinner here) and act as a kind of ink pad. You can use this printing method for a variety of things. One product ideally suited to this is making your own greetings cards. Obviously you can use different colours and different shapes to create a unique design.

LEAF PICTURES

This again will take you back to your school days. It is also a good excuse for a walk. Collect as many leaves as you can, looking for different shapes and sizes. You can do several things with them. A simple collage can be made of a pleasing design merely by arranging the leaves in whichever way you like. Alternatively you can make designs using prints of the leaves. Paint your leaves with a brush and press them down onto the paper. Leaves with pronounced veins give the best results. One other use for leaves is to make animal pictures from them, using different shapes and sizes to build up the bodies of various forms of animal life. For example, if you make a rabbit, use a large leaf for the body, a medium roundish one for the head, two long thin ones for the ears and so on. Try to create other animals such as fish or butterflies.

SPINNING PAINT

This is another personal favourite. You will need a piece of equipment which you can either make yourself or find someone to make for you. It is also available from good toy shops. You will need a small battery operated motor. You can get them from model shops (they are used to propel motor boats). You have to set this into a large, strong cardboard box or make a thin wooden one. Link the motor to the batteries incorporating an on/off switch on the outside of the box. Then, with the rotating point of your motor upwards, fix a sturdy platform to the motor. The idea is that this rotates inside the box. Now the fun starts. Fix your piece of paper onto the platform, using either Blu tac or paper clips and start the motor. Then just drop paint onto the spinning paper aiming for the centre. All you will see is a kind of blur whizzing around in the box with paint flying off in all directions covering the inside of the box. Now switch off and hey presto! Using reds and yellows will give you pictures resembling glorious sunsets. These can be good pictures in their own right or you can use them perhaps for greetings cards.

SILKSCREEN PRINTING

This is far and away the easiest, most versatile and enjoyable way of printing. It is cheap and the results are impeccable. First you need a screen printing frame which you can make yourself or buy. Craft shops sell small screen printing kits which are ideal for making greetings cards; you will rarely need anything larger and they are not expensive. However something a little larger and sturdier is useful for working with older adults as it is easier to handle. To make your own follow these instructions.

1 Make a frame with the inside measurements of 22 × 30cm (9 × 12 inches) using 3·75 × 2 mm (1·75 × 0·75 inch) timber, or as near as you can get. Hold the corner joints together using right angle, flat metal brackets, as in Figure 5.

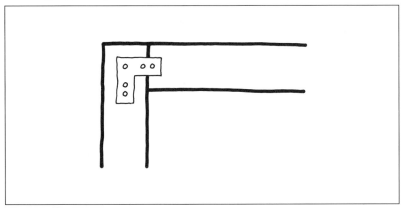

Figure 5

2 Buy half a metre (1·5 feet) of 'organdie' from any good material shop. You now stretch this over the frame, fixing it to the sides with a good stapler. Following Figure 6 staple in the order shown, stretching as you go to ensure an even tension. It needs to be taut, like a drumskin.

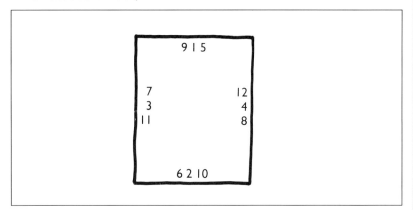

Figure 6

Work around in the same direction with a staple every 15 mm or half inch until you have covered each side and the screen is taut.

At this stage run some strong glue around the outside over the staples just to prevent any splitting of the organdie. Trim off the surplus organdie.

3 You have your screen, now you need a base for fixing it. Cut a piece of 1 cm ($\frac{1}{3}$ inch) thick plywood so that it is about 10 cm (4 inches) larger than the screen all the way around. 8 cm (3 inches) from the top screw a length of the wood you used for the frame across this base. Place the screen (organdie down) on the base, up against the crosspiece and centre it. You now need to hinge the two together. From a hardware or woodwork shop get a suitable strong hinge, but

ensure it is one where the hinge pin can be removed. This will enable you to remove the screen from the base for cleaning. You should end up with something similar to Figure 7.

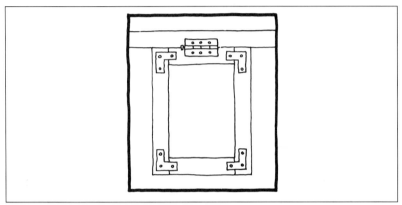

Figure 7

All you need now is a squeegee which you can buy from a craft shop — making your own is a hassle.

4 You are now ready to go into production but I suggest you mess around a bit first so that you get the hang of the basic principles involved. Eventually you will be using proper water-based screen printing ink but in order to mess about it is silly to waste ink. You can make your own using wallpaper paste and food colouring or any other coloured ink. Mix up a small amount of paste and colour it to a fairly deep hue.

5 The principle is the same as stencilling. You cut your design into a stencil. Greaseproof paper is good enough for our purposes. This is stuck to the underside of the screen using brown gummed paper. On the other side of the screen, mask the inside edges where the wood and organdie meet with more gummed paper. Place your printing paper under the screen, pour your ink or paste along the top of the

screen then draw it down along the organdie with the squeegee using a firm and steady hand. Lift the screen on its hinge and you will have a print according to the design of your stencil. The only way to learn and understand this fully is to spend time getting your hands dirty. Very soon you will be quite accomplished. Once mastered screen printing is quick to set up and easy to use and you can make your own Christmas cards, tee shirts, and so on. You can do very fine work with a greaseproof paper stencil — just draw anything and cut it out using a craft knife or scalpel. Use the talent at your local school or art college to help you if you cannot quite master it.

DOILLIES

This is quite simple and very effective and usually comes into its own around Christmas when you can make different decorations.

On a piece of paper (the size is up to you), draw a hexagon; if you want to make a lot, construct a cardboard template so that you can draw instant hexagons.

Cut your hexagon out and fold it in half, as in Figure 8, and in half again (see Figure 9).

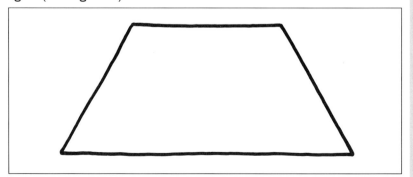

Figure 8

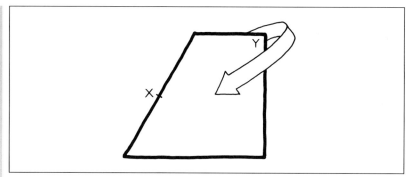

Figure 9

Mark the halfway point (x) bend point y over to meet x and crease the fold, (Figure 9).

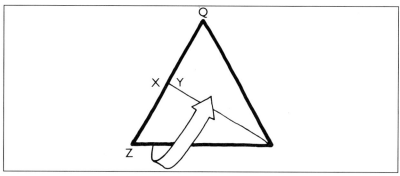

Figure 10

Now fold point z under to meet q and crease the fold, as in Figure 10.

You will end up with the shape in Figure 11.

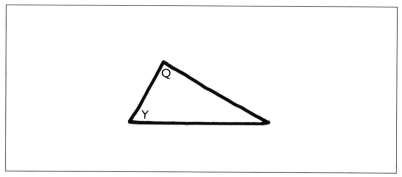

Figure 11

Now cut away at all the edges, making small incisions but leaving enough paper to give the design strength. Unfold them and you will end up with symmetrical designs resembling snowflakes. You can then make collages, cards, streamers, or hanging mobiles.

FORK FLOWERS

These are easy to do and get people's fingers moving. Thread some wool onto a fork as in Figure 12, weaving it in and out of the prongs until the fork is full, but not packed.

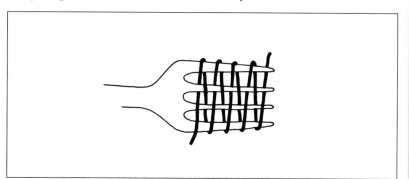

Figure 12

Then bend the end of a pipe cleaner, preferably a green one (paint your own) around the middle of all the threads (see Figure 13).

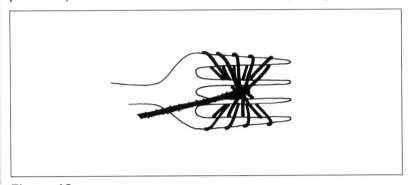

Figure 13

Pull the fork away and you are left with a flower (Figure 14).

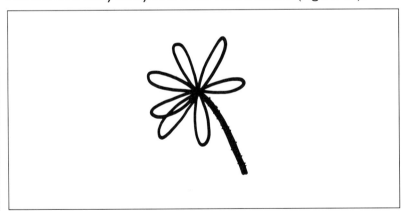

Figure 14

MOULDS

This is making statues and ornaments from plaster of paris. You can get moulds from craft shops and the resulting ornaments can then be painted. Mixing plaster of paris to the right consistency and using it before it sets is an art in itself. When dry the models can be enhanced by varnish. When fully proficient move onto mixing concrete and making those crouching cats people have in their gardens alongside garden gnomes and frogs. Moulds can be ordered from good craft suppliers. The finished product can then be painted. Fund raisers note . . . these sell very well.

DIP LAQUER

Buy tins of coloured laquer from craft shops and some pliable modelling wire to go with it. All you do to make flowers, perhaps for table decorations, is bend the wire into a petal shape, then dip it into the laquer. When dry twist the wire stems of your petals together and join in a green pipe cleaner. This is very easy and gives good results.

BASKET WEAVING

This is a traditional day centre occupation which can be either fascinating or downright boring. It is a love it or loathe it activity. It is easy to learn and with practice can give excellent results. It is good for coming back to every week and doing a little more and people often have presents in mind, which gives it a greater sense of purpose. It is also obviously good practice for manual dexterity. For those who are less dextrous, you can find plastic bases with extending 'prongs' around which raffia can be threaded.

POTTERY

This is great fun, though it can be expensive if you want to get into the realms of kilns and so forth. If you have not got a resident expert it is worth contacting your local art college for a volunteer. There are several types of modelling clay on the market which do not need firing in a kiln and these are very good. You can, for instance, make small brooches and stick them to brooch pins. A good snoop around any craft shop will give you many ideas, not just for this but for other crafts too.

DRIED FLOWERS

These are good for making greetings cards or just collages. Collect flowers, grasses and leaves having due regard for wildlife, so do not pick rare flowers and only use those where there are plenty. Dry the flowers by sandwiching them between sheets of newspaper and leaving them for a week or so with some heavy books on top. You can also make very good book marks by covering designs with clear plastic film.

DOUGH SCULPTING

This is the same as clay modelling but you use dough — edible craftwork. For the dough use three tablespoons of plain flour, one tablespoon of salt and mix it with water. Then do your modelling (you can make good wall sculptures) and bake in a cool oven (gas mark one) (275°F/140°C) for about an hour; leave to cool. You can colour the results with felt pens and then varnish them. Another possibility is using pastry cutters; you could make Christmas tree decorations from the more interesting shapes.

PAPIER MÂCHÉ

Another cheap and messy modelling medium but one that is quite versatile. The best kind of paper to use is newsprint, which can be mixed with cold water wallpaper paste. There are two basic methods. The first is to use the mâché like clay and just sculpt with it. The second is to layer pieces of soaked paper around a mould. An example would be making a dish by layering the paper to the required thickness around the outside of a pottery bowl.

PAPIER MÂCHÉ CHRISTMAS BAUBLES

Using oranges, cover them with strips of newspaper stuck down with wallpaper paste — about six layers deep or so, enough to give it strength. Leave for a day to dry thoroughly, then cut in half with a scalpel. The two halves should come away from the orange fairly easily. Use tape or papier mâché strips to put the two halves together again. Now make a loop around a knife handle with a piece of wire and twist it, then bend the ends at right angles to the loop, as in Figure 15.

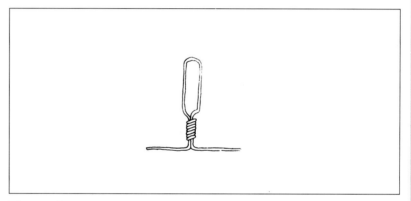

Figure 15

Tape this to the top of the ball and you are ready to be creative.

Using small thin strips of paper cut from colour magazines, collage over the whole surface, smoothing it out as you go.

Now dream up weird and wonderful designs, such as animals or plants.

When you have finished varnish the whole thing several times. The results are very pleasing. For large rooms you can make unusual decorations by using papier mâché over a balloon. Again collage them and varnish. These are good because they are larger and so easier to handle and there is no messing around with scalpels and bits of wire. A group could make them, different people working on the various stages: cutting, pasting, collage choosing, sticking and varnishing.

PINBOARDS

This is good for manual skills and hand/eye co-ordination. You can buy books of designs and make your own boards from plywood, hammering the pins in position. You can make some very pleasing designs and once you have got the hang of it this activity becomes quite easy. The pinboards can be used over and over again, you don't have to keep them for ever.

MARBLING

This is easy to do, good fun and produces interesting results. You can get marbling colours from craft shops. Simply half fill a large square washing up bowl with water and drop the colours onto the surface. Comb, blow or swirl the colours whichever way takes your fancy. Place a piece of paper onto the surface and lift it off again. This makes excellent wrapping paper for small gifts, or covers for books.

DO IT YOURSELF

You can buy simple ready-cut wood kits of, for example, bird boxes which you just need to sand, glue and nail, then varnish. This is easily accomplished and looks very good. Good craft suppliers will have other kits, like spice racks. Eventually move onto greater heights — cut your own wood, design your own simple book racks and book ends, erect full scale replicas of medieval tithe barns, even build a yacht!

TAPESTRY

Kits are obviously very good, but do not forget you can paint on plain canvas and work your own design. You can now get sheets of plastic canvas which are easier to work (larger holes) for those without nimble fingers, or those not wishing to go cross-eyed finding the hole. These can be cut to any shape. One excellent use is to cut small shapes and work them in bright colours for Christmas tree decorations.

Section F

PERCEPTION & ORIENTATION

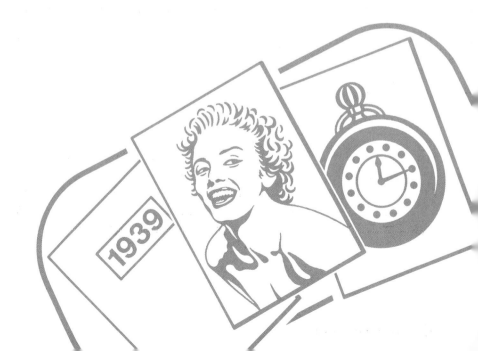

The games and exercises described here are some of the most useful and most enjoyable you will come across. They are easy to organise and the degree of difficulty can be varied enormously. Some of the interaction games already described would fall into this category as well.

Besides being good fun for the group these exercises, like so many others, can highlight cognitive deficits, but more obviously they can bring to light any sensory deficits that might otherwise be missed.

SENSORY DEFICIT

Obviously where there is a sensory deficit, one should focus upon the remaining senses. People suffering from blindness or partial loss of sight often have a very keen sense of hearing, touch, smell and taste. Whilst hearing is the sense often used to compensate for loss of vision, touch is also very important, but is often avoided by the sighted for reasons of social 'taboo' or custom. Cultural norms and values must be respected but be aware of the potential of touch. The way something feels creates an image in the mind. Close your eyes and put your hand on the telephone and instantly you have it in your mind. If the buttons have raised numbers or braille then away you go.

Explaining clearly all that you do and all that is happening in the group is important. Taking, for example, a blind lady from a hospital ward to the x-ray department in a wheelchair would be a frightening experience if no explanation were given. Blindfolding each other and leading your partner around your familiar workplace will give you an understanding of why explanations are crucial.

In groups always try and have a co-worker sitting next to anybody with a visual handicap so that they can constantly update them as to what is going on. Describe in detail any visual aids. We have a lovely lady who is totally blind, yet who loves the slide groups we hold. One of us always sits with her and describes the slide in fine detail, which is a springboard for her to talk about the subject in hand. So always bear in mind that with a little help and adjustment a poorly sighted person can participate in and enjoy most of the groups. Groups based on the other senses can give blind people a chance to excel and provide the rest of the group with a chance to reappraise the skills of the blind.

Again, with hearing difficulties it is most important to have someone sitting next to the client but facing them slightly so they can explain what is happening. This gives the client a chance to lip read. With hearing aids you may find that the batteries are flat, the tubes are clogged with wax, they emit a high pitched whistle or are on the wrong setting. Always check hearing aids for these things. The loop system is of benefit here if used in conjunction with a microphone. It makes the speaker's voice much clearer through the hearing aid.

SIGHT AND VISUAL GAMES

'WHITE POWDERY STUFF'

Find half a dozen or so saucers and place in them similar white powders such as sugar, salt, washing powder, talcum powder, flour

or

coconut, rice, sago, tapioca, oatmeal.

The object then is to differentiate visually between the contents.

ACTIVITIES

ILLUSIONS

There are many illusions that you can find in and copy from books. The old man/young girl one is the obvious one that springs to mind. But others are . . .

Who is the tallest?

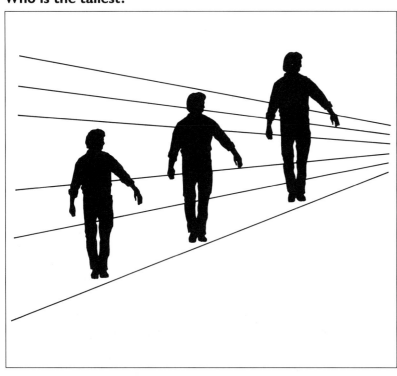

Which lines are the longest?

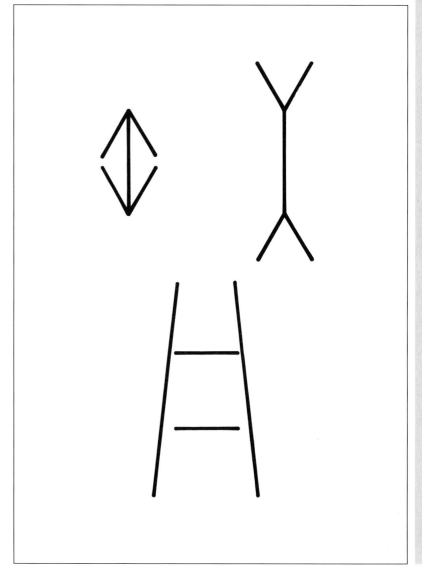

Which black dot is bigger?

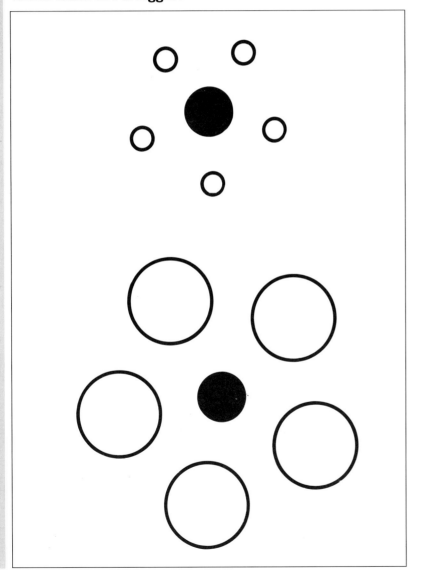

Old or young?

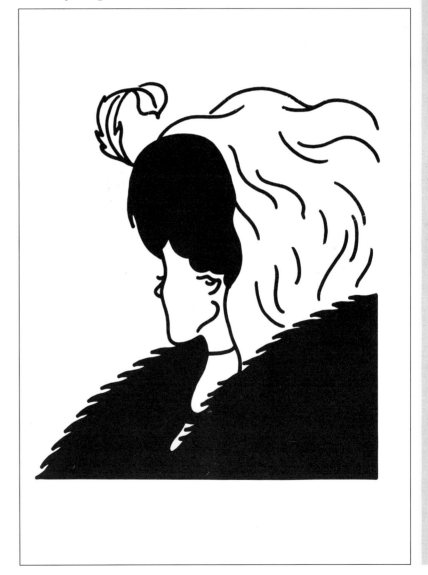

What do you see?

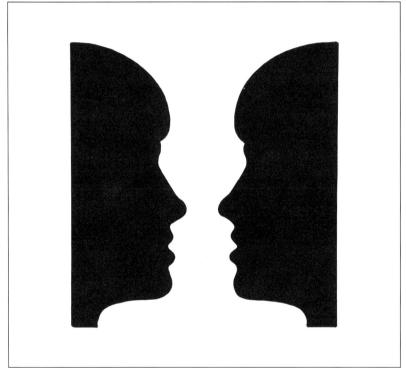

Rabbit or duck?

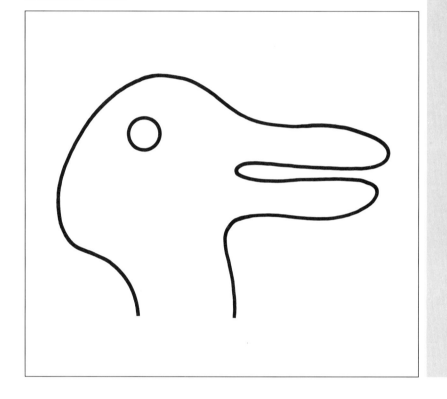

What is it?

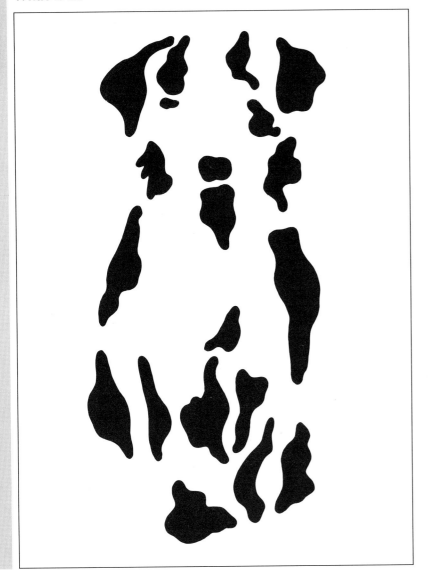

Which is the front?

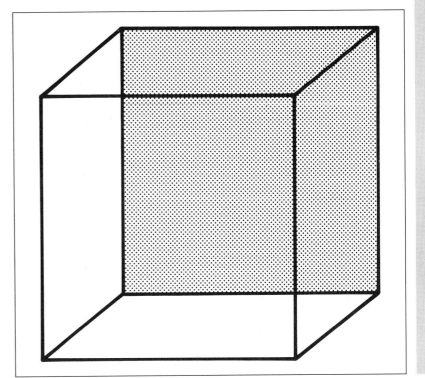

?

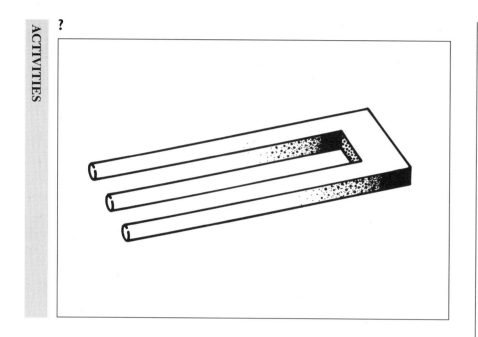

Straight or not!

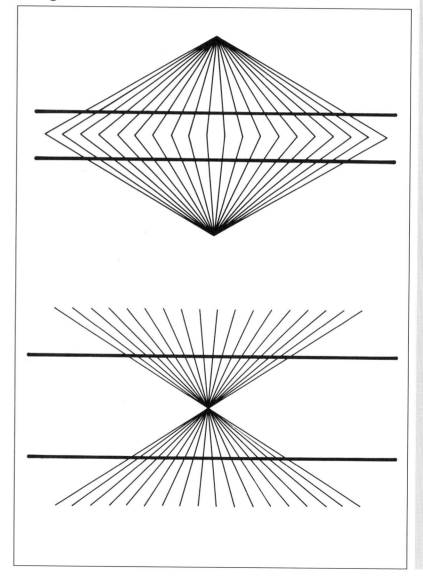

WHAT IS IT? (I)

What you need are five cards with gradually increasing holes in them. The top card has a hole about 5 cm (2 inches) in diameter, the bottom one about 20 cm (8 inches) in diameter. Place them over a picture, small holes last, so that when you hold it up to the group they can only see a small part of the picture. The idea is that they try and guess what it is. You gradually remove the cards so they see a little more of the picture until someone guesses it, and then reveal it. The degree of difficulty can be varied widely and so it can be used for all levels of ability.

You need good, large, clear pictures such as a tree, a baby's face, a bread loaf, a close up of a cat's face. As well as being large they should preferably be in colour. Many such pictures can be found in a wide variety of magazines.

A good variation is to use famous faces pictures, gradually revealing more and seeing how long it takes to guess who; or you can use such subjects as places, wildlife, and so on.

WHAT IS IT? (2)

This is similar to the TV programme 'Antiques Roadshow' but instead of antiques you present unusual objects which can be passed around. This can be great fun with people trying to guess what it is and for what purpose it might be used.

Things we can use are:

Corner protectors (things you put on the corners of tables to protect young children who may fall against them)

Unusual tools — such as a spark plug remover

A hand held slide viewer

A cigarette roller

One of those plastic balls in which you put washing powder.

UNUSUAL ANGLES

These are pictures of everyday objects taken from unusual angles or from very close range. The object is obviously to guess what it is. You can buy them or photograph your own. You can either use a black and white film and blow them up on a photocopier, or you can make slides and show them on the wall. Using slides makes it more of an event. Have one slide of the close up followed by one revealing the object as it is usually seen.

POSTCARD PUZZLES

This is meant for small groups of two, three, or four. Cut up several postcards into four or five odd-shaped pieces and mix them all up. Give each person, sitting around a table, one piece from a different postcard. They now have to find the other three or four pieces and make up the picture. It is a simple jigsaw but it can be made more difficult by cutting the postcards into smaller pieces or using postcards of the same view but cut up slightly differently.

SILHOUETTES

Using your famous faces and pictures of animals or anything else you wish, make a tracing of the outlines or profiles. Transfer these onto sheets of paper and black them in.

ART APPRECIATION

This is not so much to do with perception but our appreciation of what we perceive.

For this you will need a collection of pictures of famous and not so famous works of art. You can cut them from magazines, buy postcards and cheap prints. You can also buy slides of works of art from most art galleries. Each picture should be discussed in turn and each participant should be encouraged to give an opinion. Do you like it? Would you buy it? Would you want to look at it on your wall every morning? Abstract works should be included as these can stimulate much discussion of styles and personal tastes.

Following the discussion hold a mock auction whereby you sell off the pictures to the highest bidder according to taste. This should stimulate discussion as to the value we place on works of art as compared to other things.

CHILDREN'S WORK

Ask a local school to supply you regularly with a selection of art work done by the children. Ask the teacher to put the name, age and subject on the back of each one. These can be shown to the group for appreciation and discussion. This can also be a useful reminiscing session about our own school days. It is also interesting to try and guess the age of the artist, what details can be picked out and whether a boy or girl painted it.

SOUND

TAPES

There are various tapes you can buy commercially or make yourself.

Animal sounds are good and much harder than you would think. You can discuss the purpose behind the animal sound. Does it sound happy or frightened, are they calling to each other or just yelling for the sake of it?

You can also buy sound effect records which are very good. They have things like a door creaking, a storm, a car being started up.

Any good record dealer should be able to help you out and order one for you — the BBC one is especially useful here. Another good variant is a tape of the sounds of different musical instruments. You could ask your local school or music college to make one for you.

LIVE SOUNDS

You can avoid using tapes by making everyday sounds 'live'. From behind a screen you can make various noises for the members to guess, such as:

pouring water	shuffling cards
striking a match	rattling money or keys
cracking an egg	rustling leaves

flicking through a newspaper, and so on.

SOUND GUESS

Fill some small containers which are not see-through with various things like water, sugar, drawing pins, rice, buttons, a rubber. There are lots of things you can use which make different sounds. These are then passed around the group for each member to shake and guess what is inside.

BLIND QUOTE

See *Interaction Groups*.

TOUCH

PILLOW GUESS

This is basically identifying something by touch, without having to blindfold everybody.

Place an everyday object in the pillow case and and tie it up, then pass it around the group getting them to have a good feel, to describe it and say what they think it is. All sorts of factors like shape, size and weight come into play so there are several clues. The sort of things you can use are a telephone, clock, cheese grater, kettle, potato scoop, top hat, packet of cream crackers, hairdryer, golf ball, pen, reel of cotton, mouth organ.

A variation is to use natural objects like twigs, dried leaves, pebbles, conkers; or everyday objects like newspaper, drinks cans and the like. This has the bonus of being a sound exercise as well. Scrunch it and bang it; what does it sound like?

Other variations are to have several pillow cases with similar objects inside; they put their hand in and feel, for example, different types of fabric — silk, hessian, cotton. Another alternative is different types of fruit and vegetables. The variations here are legion, given a bit of imagination.

THE LAYING ON OF HANDS

This is one for a group which has been running for some time and where the members are fairly familiar with each other.

Taking it in turns, ask one of the members to sit on a chair in the middle of the group and wear a blindfold. Once in the hot spot ask them to hold their hands out in front of them palms uppermost. Ask the other group members to stand up and walk around and then sit down again except for one of them who places their hands palm down on those of our guinea pig.

They then have to say who they think it is and why. There are several clues including size, lightness of touch, male or female.

FACE GUESS

See *Interaction Groups*.

Again, this is only for a group that is fairly well developed and who know each other well enough.

SMELL

Apart from testing our sense of smell this is great fun. You will find that ability here varies enormously. You need appropriate containers whereby you cannot see inside but can smell the substance. I used urine specimen bottles painted white with holes punched in the metal top. The containers are passed around for comment.

Useful substances are: pine, mustard, shampoo, tea leaves, cigar tobacco, horseradish sauce, herbs, onion, vinegar, spices, perfume, lemon juice, curry powder, orange oil, ginger, a hard boiled egg, cloves, mint and malt.

Just to keep everyone on their toes I usually pass one around that has not got anything in it!

You can supply clues like — "Is it pleasant or unpleasant?", "Is it to do with food?", "Would you dab it behind your ears or put it on your chips?"

You can also try and capture smells which give an image of a place or situation. What is that smell you always get in a hospital? I've never found it, but a fresh fabric plaster comes close — it must be disinfectant. Freshly-cut grass is like that smell of cleanness you get after rain. Ask the group to suggest ideas for smells.

TASTE

This is a bit trickier to organise unless you make everybody sit around wearing blindfolds.

Otherwise you can use flavoured colourless liquids — for instance sugar, salt, lemon, vinegar, gin, water, lemonade, mineral water and tonic water.

You can taste powders as well; give everybody a spoon with which to sample sugar, salt, custard powder, flour, coconut, ground rice, sherbet, powdered milk, banana, strawberry and chocolate flavoured build-ups, powdered egg, powdered potato and so on.

It is useful though to supply everybody with a large glass of water to clear the palate and a bucket in case they do not wish to swallow.

These are not specifically for people with poor memories, indeed they often should not be used with such people, as they can be frustratingly difficult. As with the other groups you must decide what is appropriate for which particular clients.

I WENT TO MARKET

Most people will be familiar with this. With the group sitting in a close circle so that everyone can hear, someone starts by saying "I went to market and bought a pound of tomatoes", the next person adds an extra item and so on and so on until there are just too many items to remember them all.

It is useful for the leader to scribble the items down as they are said so that you can go through the list afterwards, because the leader will inevitably be unable to remember them.

KIM'S GAME

Otherwise called *Memory Tray*.

Place ten or so (depending upon group size and ability) objects which are easily recognisable on a tray and cover it with a pillow case or towel. Explain to the group that you are going to uncover the tray for a while, then cover it again and you want them to then remember what was on it. A slow count of ten seems about right; invite the members to get close and have a good look.

Then when the tray is covered ask them to brainstorm the objects and write them upon the blackboard as they are shouted out.

Then do another group exercise for a quarter or half an hour having put the tray to one side. When you have finished ask again what was on the tray.

If it starts getting too easy then increase the number of items on the tray or reduce the amount of time it is uncovered.

Be careful to use recognisable items for the age group — a bottle of Tippex might be to hand but it is not necessarily an object known to our clients. An interesting alternative is to show a tray of objects, then remove one or two and show the tray again and ask which objects have been removed.

STRANGERS

Pre-arrange with a colleague who is not well known to the group to walk into the room, pick something up and walk out again. Get them to do this halfway through a group, then at the end ask the members if they can recall:

1 What the person did
2 Height
3 Clothes
4 Colour of hair and style
5 Any other distinguishing features.

Sharing reminiscences, looking at pictures of the old days and how things have changed is a great social event. We have all said "It's not like it used to be" more times than we would care to remember. We all have many memories and a huge back catalogue of experiences, and by sharing reminiscences with elderly people we can learn what they found to be of value and comfort in their earlier days, what their interests were and what made them tick. It is our past which gives us our identity and makes us unique and distinct from others. By exploring significant past events we reinforce our distinctiveness and so maintain our identity. Participants in these groups contribute something which is uniquely theirs, and attention and encouragement from the therapists and other group members will greatly boost confidence and self-esteem. The clients with their wealth of experience are the experts here.

Reminiscence is important for most of us . . . that is why we take photos, it is not a question of living in the past. The benefits can be broadly categorised thus:

1 Self Identity

Reminiscence as we have said underlines the uniqueness of our experience. Recalling past experiences helps maintain our self-identity and gives us a place in history.

2 Self-Esteem

Giving accounts of what you have done and receiving attention boosts your ego, it makes you feel that you have something valid to say. If others then have similar reminiscences it gives you a feeling of belonging and overcomes the sense of isolation that old age can bring.

3 Life Review

In old age it is often important to evaluate your life, take stock and go over your achievements, traumas, failures and good times. It can give you a sense of satisfaction and perspective, and enable you to come to terms with life's disappointments.

4 Fun

Chewing the fat about old times is simply just good fun. Much social interaction can be stimulated by imaginative and lively reminiscence events.

SOME CONSIDERATIONS

Whilst reminiscence is usually viewed as fun it can be just the opposite. In a group situation there may be much animation and sharing but there may also be those who do not share this enthusiasm, for good reasons. For example, the war years were a devastating experience that many may well not wish to explore again. For other people, they may not be able to reminisce because of the stark and unpleasant contrast between a rich and satisfying past and a lonely, deprived present. Placing the reminiscence within an individualised plan of care and obtaining a thorough history from those who know your clients well should help to avoid this mistake.

Similarly the age span of an elderly client group can be surprisingly large and this needs to be taken into account. Using the war as an example again, in just the space of ten years between people aged 60 to those aged 70 there will be a large range of experiences from the child who vaguely remembers the disruption in home life to those who actively served and lost family and friends.

Nor is it just the major historical events which should dominate reminiscence. It is the peculiarities and idiosyncrasies of everyday life which make up the largest proportion of our experience. I can personally recollect almost nothing of the politics of the era when I was ten years old without being heavily prompted. The only major event I can recall is the 1966 World Cup. However I can recall my school, the cigarette card games in the playground, conkers, my first pair of football boots, my friends, their toys, being confined to the garden for being home late, the meals we had, our weekends and Sunday walks. These are what shaped me as a person and make me unique. Using such personal histories we can steer reminiscence away from the major events and try and concentrate on the uniquely personal, often humdrum, but distinctive details that make our lives so varied.

As with other groupwork areas, imagination and enthusiasm can turn reminiscence into an art form. In its most basic form it usually involves the passing around of pictures as triggers to recollection and discussion. We have five senses though and all can be engaged to stimulate reminiscence. You can recreate living scenarios such as tea dances and pub singalongs by simply readjusting the furniture. In this way reminiscence sessions can become major events. Dressing up and baking from the old recipes can all add to the sense of atmosphere and period.

IDEAS FOR REMINISCENCE

Scrapbook
For many of the categories listed below making a scrapbook is by far the most effective and versatile reminiscence tool. By far your best source of pictures are the magazines from Sunday papers and any others you can scrounge covering the particular subject area. Once made they are a permanent resource.

Natural History
A scrapbook of animals and plants of the countryside can easily be made from magazines. Ask your local natural history society for help here and you may even get speakers and slide shows.

Everyday Objects
Pictures for recognition can be obtained from magazines and shopping catalogues. A quick trip round the shops for product brochures will help. Almost anything is included here; watches, irons, cheese, cars, toys, jewellery, clothes, and household knick-knacks. Remember, though, try and get hold of the real thing so that clients can handle them and demonstrate their use.

Seasons
Make collages of seasons and other yearly events such as Christmas and Easter. See the art and craft chapter for a list of themes.

Old Postcards and Books
Old postcards can be expensive, but you can now get sets of reproduced cards of yesteryear. Apart from postcards, travel books with large colour pictures are still surprisingly cheap, as are (even more so) old film year books with large colour prints of yesterday's stars.

Cigarette Cards
They do not produce these anymore. However, they are available

at collectors' fairs and you can still get bargains. Look out especially for film stars series.

Books

Not as daft as it sounds, you can get some good reminiscence books. For example, there is a good book of the best from 'Picture Post'. There are also many good books of the war years, animals and most other categories. Many towns do 'then and now' type books from old postcards.

Famous People

Pictures of famous people from yesteryear are sure memory joggers and one picture can spark off a whole series of associations.

Gardening

Again using pictures and tools as props this subject can trigger many memories. Even those who did not engage in other hobbies may well have tended a garden or even kept an allotment. Using real flowers as props stimulates the senses. You can even buy a selection of fruits and discuss if they taste as good as they used to.

Shopping

The interaction game 'what price is it?' can be used as a trigger to talk about how things have changed; the prices, the styles, the shops. A trip to a local superstore might raise a few eyebrows. Where are the penny woodbines? Whatever happened to the ten bob note?

Occupations

You can use pictures of people in different uniforms or performing various tasks. Try and use props such as a policeman's helmet, pick axe, saw, surgeon's face mask. Many of the old trades and jobs have now died out and these can be explored using pictures as triggers, for example, a bus conductor, wheelwright, blacksmith.

Sport

This can be an excuse for another scrapbook and a few games. School sports days can be explored and any trophies we won, or nearly won! Teams we supported and childhood heroes can also be discussed.

Transport

Another excuse for a scrapbook!

Places

There are several areas to concentrate on here. Local landmarks, landmarks from Britain and the wider world. Travel agents are a good source of pictures here.

Slides

See chapter on slides.

Videos

You are by now aware that you can now get videos of individual years and decades. So put the kettle on and sit back with the remote control so that you can pause, rewind and stop at appropriate points for discussion. You can also, of course, recreate the cinema, complete with usherette and torch, intervals and choc ices. There are many old 'classic' films now available on video, which you can advertise in advance, building up to the 'showing' when you rearrange the room accordingly.

Weather

This is a perennial theme. Did it really snow more when we were children? Recollected storms, floods and heat waves can all be useful triggers and can be backed up with newspaper accounts from the time. Many local papers have a small 10, 20 and 30 years ago section. The local museum may well have archive material relating to local occurrences.

Holidays

Inextricably linked with the weather, holidays usually generate much discussion. They were usually so enjoyable as small children that they became well embedded in the memory. Many will have visited the same local resort, pictures of which can be passed around. You can even go there on a reminiscence trip. Beware though, some people could not afford to go on holiday and may not want reminding of the fact.

Food

Again pictures from magazines can be useful prompters as to what we used to eat. How people coped with rationing and what used to be a treat or a luxury can all be focused upon. You can get 'old' recipes from books and your clients can organise baking sessions.

Fashion

Find some old pictures to contrast with modern styles. This usually raises a few eyebrows. Props can be tried to add some fun, especially hats and shoes.

Royalty

This is fairly obvious and another excuse for a scrapbook. It is also good for that strange reason that we can nearly always remember where we were at times of national and international importance, for instance, the Coronation and Arsenal winning the double!

Hobbies

Also included here are arts and crafts. What we were good (or lousy) at, what we made at school, what our interests were before our responsibilities got in the way and why we let them.

Objet D'Antique

This is a good excuse for getting old objects, not necessarily antique, and passing them around, having a look and feel and reminding ourselves for what they were used. If possible have modern counterparts as well with which to contrast them. If you cannot get the real thing start collecting pictures of 'then and now' contrasts, such as fashion, cars, household and kitchen items. Ask your local museum for help.

War

One is tempted to say enough is enough, must we drone on about this evil period. Well, yes, our clients lived through it, we did not and the effect it had on their lives must have been profound beyond our comprehension. Use props where possible, such as ration book, gas mask, ARP hat.

There is nothing stopping you relating their experiences to moral issues, discussing man's stupidity and inhumanity, they have first-hand experience of these sad human traits. But remember some people may rightly not want to be reminded. Pacifism is not a modern concept.

Childhood and Family Life

This opens the gates to many different areas; the radio, your first television, schooldays, children's games, pocket money, household chores. Try and get old photos to use, school photos, family holidays and so on. Bring out your old school reports if you dare; this should stimulate some feelings such as how it felt as you handed it to your parents.

Music

Refer to the music chapter and be prepared to singalong. Have pictures of the old favourites to back it up. Recreate tea-dances and the feeling of the music hall or the pub 'tap room' singalong.

Personal History Boards

These are for use on bedside lockers and the like. Basically they are a collage comprising important aspects of a person's life — photos of self and families, and pets, postcards of favourite holiday spots, pictures of hobbies, club badges, ties, bus passes, member-ship cards and so forth. All these can help with self identity and trigger the recollection of 'who I am'.

Collage

In the art and craft chapter you will find a list of collage themes, most of which can be used for individual and group reminiscence sessions. Using any theme, a collage is a useful way of focusing a group.

Museums

Many museums now have recreations of houses, rooms and shops 'as they were'. These are probably the closest you will get to the real thing. Here is a vast wealth of reminiscence material and it is worth asking the curator if they can organise a 'hands-on' session for your group.

REALITY ORIENTATION

There has been much written about reality orientation (RO) and indeed there is much that needs to be said about it. It is often too heavily relied upon and inappropriately used and often wrongly dismissed as valueless. Before we enter into the debate let us just say that there is a use and a misuse for everything; the golden rule, as in all good group-work, is aiming what you do at the right level for the particular group of clients with whom you are dealing. Between being moderately and severely demented lie an infinite number of degrees. You must, and you can, know where your clients are at, and aim your intervention at that level; if you do not you will either frustrate or ridicule and you could insult and cause severe distress.

Basically then, reality orientation aims to help people retain basic information regarding self and others and their orientation in time and place. It seeks to enable the short-term memory.

Reality orientation has traditionally centred around an RO board which indicates the day, date, place, weather, staff members on duty and the day's events. The board is a link between the two faces of RO, firstly, 24-hour RO and secondly group and individual sessions. Whilst acknowledging that we cannot reverse dementia it is widely agreed that we may be able to slow down the disabling effects of the underlying disease. Twenty-four hour RO is an ongoing process used in all interaction throughout the day. It involves always saying the client's and your own name, reminding people of their surroundings and constantly reinforcing what is happening — a bit like a running commentary on the daily routine. It is not specifically done in the hope of the client remembering but as a constant source of reference of information that is of value, as if you are constantly allaying fears and putting people at ease. That is where the loo is, this is where we are in the day, what meal is coming, who that young man is to whom you are talking. Again, knowing your client tells you how specific to be or not. For example, "here, try using your fork", may be OK to some, but to others who have forgotten what a fork is for, then you need to step up a gear and say "this is a fork, you can use it to help you eat, like this".

Another aspect of 24-hour RO is the widespread use of labelling. 'John's bed', 'toilet', 'kitchen', . . . again, the words may be meaningless to some so back them up by using pictures. Similarly if you are talking about the weather do not just stop at verbal description, take people out and let them experience it; point out the wet roads, trees bending in the wind, the sound of the rain and the feel of the snow.

Always try to foresee failure in order to prevent it. If someone's memory is so bad they will not be able to answer, then provide the answer with the question, do not leave them frustrated and guessing. For example, instead of asking "what is the weather like?", try "it is a lovely sunny day today, isn't it?"

More formally, RO takes place in groups where various themes are discussed. Attention and concentration span is usually fairly brief so the group should be short and concise. Such groups should be friendly and fun — always start with the kettle! Name badges and introductions are useful and can be reinforced early on over a cup of tea and a swift explanation of the RO board before concentrating on the theme. The groups should be small, regular and frequent and members should be of similar levels of ability. Foreknowledge of your clients is invaluable in making the sessions more pertinent . . . get to know what jobs they had, hobbies, where they lived. In this way you will get good interaction and shared activity at the right pitch personalized for that particular group's members.

ORIENTATION, VALIDATION, RESOLUTION

Reality orientation has recently been fairly heavily criticised for 'blanket application'. Who cares what day it is? It is pointless reinforcing that which will be immediately forgotten. Such criticisms arise from an erroneous comparison with the increasing use of validation therapy and more recently resolution therapy. People have tended to see a dichotomy between the therapies . . . validation versus orientation. This is an error as, correctly used, the two should complement each other. However, the fact remains that if memory loss is so severe then it is pointless reminding people of such matters as the day and date.

We must acknowledge that there comes a time when the dementia has progressed so far that reorientation is impossible and fruitless. Continuing its use after this point is reached is annoying to the client and frustrating. If any insight is retained we are merely reminding them of how hopeless their memory is.

Countering this argument, when the point of virtually no useful memory is reached, appropriate RO can still be a means of structuring reassuring social contact in the 'here and now'. Having to exist in the 'here and now' without any real comprehension of it must be a profoundly frightening experience. Reality orientation recognises this fact and urges us to explore the underlying feelings and emotions of the statements of those so apparently out of touch with our 'here and now' reality.

Validation therapy is applicable only in mild or reversible confusional states of psychological origin. It necessitates an ability to reflect on past life events and requires cognitive skills which are severely diminished in the later stages of organic dementias such as Alzheimer's disease and multi-infarct dementia.

Resolution therapy, as described by Stokes and Goudie (1990) takes the concept of exploring underlying feelings further and is a valuable counselling tool for those suffering organic dementing illnesses. Resolution assumes that whatever the patient says NOW is the reality for them and it is pointless to try and change it. We should try and understand it. It has deep and real meaning for them even though it may be fantasy for us. Such 'realities' are often focused on past life events. It is common for very elderly clients to speak of their parents as being alive. Hence the 88-year-old lady becomes a teenager — "Mum'll kill me if I don't get home soon, I've got to go to the shops for her." What we can do is help the client explore these experiences, try and understand their reality. Thus resolution therapy does not allow our reality to correct theirs, it accepts it as being valid. We should answer "That must be worrying, what do you have to get from the shop"; NOT, "you're 83 years old, your mother's dead, my name's Danny and it's raining outside". Instead, join in and talk about getting home late, explore the fear and excitement as if you were there, are there and have been in exactly the same boat, because you have.

There is nothing wrong with colluding with an elderly demented client, as long as you are not using it as a means to an end, so as to avoid confrontation, rather than recognizing it and using it to resolve the conflict it signifies. The key is to do whatever it takes to make that person feel valid, accepted, understood and happy.

There has, unfortunately, been much written about validation therapy, building it up out of all proportion, such as promoting it as a means of helping the client to 'resolve unfinished historical emotional conflicts'. In contrast, the basic approach of resolution therapy resolves no such conflicts but emphasizes the reality, impoverished ability to communicate and most importantly the dignity of the individual. The therapist tries to experience acceptance of whatever the client is feeling or expressing at the time and helps the client express that particular emotion or feeling by seeking to understand it, and hence helps them deal with it.

The 'relationship' you develop is the therapy which aims to restore the client's self-esteem and role on their terms without being judgemental. We have seen already that many confused elderly people with profound memory loss cope with their confusion and disorientation by seemingly reverting to a previous meaningful reality. In organic dementia this is not a conscious decision but the result of long-term memory becoming the major point of reference, that is, the past becomes the present reality. This can be said to inadvertently enable them to escape from the stress of the unfamiliar and bewildering present reality. Their behaviour in doing so can appear quite bizarre and they can be judged wrongly against the standards of behaviour of the reality of our present society or situation, which is no longer, of course, meaningful to them.

Leonard Babins (1986) describes it brilliantly, "they are coping in the most adaptive manner possible given their set of life experiences. Some patients withdraw, retreating to their own inner cosmos, or constantly dozing off to avoid reality, whilst others may resist or fight their helplessness by aggressive behaviour such as yelling and screaming, resulting in their being tranquillized and restrained." There is much we can learn from this.

RESEARCH

What help are we given by research to suggest whether reality orientation actually works? There is a large body of writing on reality orientation, notably Holden and Woods (1988), and more recently much discussion of validation therapy. Despite much misinterpretation, validation therapy does not condemn the value of RO but upholds it. However, most clinical trials and studies of individual RO programmes tend to be overwhelmingly inconclusive.

What I will suggest from the research is that it is not so much the content of RO which is the most important therapeutic factor, but merely the engaging of people in meaningful activities. That inactivity is a factor in the decline of mental and social functioning should be obvious, yet the report *Time for Action* (1982) claims that "too many old people in hospitals, day centres and nursing homes, still spend the last years of their lives sitting in chairs with nothing to do but sleep". With this in mind, any purposeful activity with elderly people could be said to be beneficial.

Argyle (1967) reminds us of one general psychological principle which is often overlooked, namely, "the detailed techniques used by therapists are less important than the therapist's own personality and more general social skills". What he is saying is that the single most important factor in therapy is the kind of relationship the therapist can develop.

We could argue then that it is not the RO techniques which are important but the bringing together of people by a skilled therapist having 'Argyle's qualities'. These qualities are, to all intents and purposes, those which Rogers (1965) identifies as being necessary for a counselling relationship; unconditional positive regard, genuineness, warmth and empathy.

Reality orientation or any other groupwork with elderly people will be largely ineffective without relationships based on these concepts. Linked with the relationship we develop with our clients is our attitude towards them and more specifically our expectations of them. Fuchs (1968) in the field of education argues "that preconceived beliefs about the capabilities of children based on their social background makes failures inevitable because expectations of failure affect instruction".

A self-fulfilling prophecy is in operation here whereby low expectations lead to low achievement which is then blamed on the child's background. This is a sociological fact well known to the proponents of labelling theory. Dementia is a label which implies low cognitive ability, poor recall, memory, concentration and so on; and hence low achievement; thus our expectations may well be subconsciously already defined at a very low level.

Given routine, rigid day/time/date/place reality orientation by uncommitted staff, sticking to this basic format, who have low expectations of their clients' capacity for success, and little faith in the techniques they use, then these expectations will inevitably be confirmed. What is needed is a far more stimulating groupwork scenario by committed staff whose expectations of their charges are optimistic.

This is not a criticism of RO but a criticism of the way it has been used. It is also usually unsuccessful because we do not correctly assess the needs and capabilities of those on whom we use it.

It is pertinent, at this point, to look briefly at some more specific studies and summarise their findings.

Holden and Woods (1982) looked at 19 trials of fairly rigid RO groups in the context of a 24-hour RO environment. Their findings were inconclusive, for while they found that verbal orientation improved, behaviour change was hardly indicated. Woods (1979) concluded that it was the attention given to clients over their whole day which was of greater benefit in improving orientation than formal RO sessions. Brook et al (1975) argue that RO is only effective where the therapists actively participate. Mere exposure to a stimulating environment is not enough to produce sustained improvement. Reinforcement and positive encouragement by the therapist is the most significant factor in stimulating change.

Merchant and Saxby (1981) argue that RO is a restimulation of awareness of the outside world and that this should be part of good nursing practice anyway. With the only mildly confused, they recorded improvements in 'awareness of others' and the ability to hold a conversation. This is somewhat backed up by Burton (1982), who upholds the orientation value of RO, but criticises the appropriateness of some of the people to whom it is applied. He cites studies by Zepelin et al (1981) which indicate that whilst improvements in orientation occurred they seldom lingered for any period of time.

Knowing what we do of the biological forces at work in dementia we should not expect any lingering gain anyway and Burton (1982) rightly concludes that whilst RO can hold back some of the effects of dementia, more importantly, it improves the quality of life.

RESOLUTION

Whilst validation therapy urges us to orient ourselves to our clients' reality, we as therapists need to keep a clear head. Where validation suggests that the client may be trying to resolve 'unfinished emotional conflicts', resolution therapy has no such lofty claims.

Whilst RO recognizes underlying emotions and hidden meanings it is essentially a memory therapy. It is not a counselling technique for exploring meanings and feelings.

Validation therapy is correct in that it too recognizes such meanings and feelings within confusion and seeks to engage the confused person on these terms. It encourages the exploration of meanings but roots them in past emotional turmoil which it assumes still needs 'working through'. This is only of value in 'pseudo-dementias' as in depression. Resolution therapy on the other hand does provide a technique of interacting with and counselling those suffering from organic dementias. Confusion here is seen as an attempt to make sense of, or a reaction to, our strange 'here and now' reality. The verbal communications of the confused are seen as attempts to express need. These 'confused' messages have both concealed meanings and underlying feelings attached. The aim of resolution is to seek them out, explore them and, it is hoped, resolve them.

The message may be confused but the meaning and feeling are very real. Left unresolved, such messages are all too easily written off as difficult behaviour. To illustrate the usefulness of resolution therapy I give the example of an elderly retired school teacher. She has been severely demented for several years and spends much of her time on the ward back in the role of a teacher, continually inspecting, rebuking, marshalling and rearranging. "Now sit down; now look, nobody is doing anything until you all sit still." With this she will glare with menacing authority at anybody who so much as moves a muscle. At other times she is constantly moving and turning furniture (back to its proper position, in her eyes) or tapping on the wall (putting up notices) or counting the lines in a copy of *Woman's Own* (doing her paperwork or marking essays). Her husband knows she is happy on the ward because when he visits she says to him, "this is a very good college dear". To redirect her in these activities leads to extreme frustration, anger, aggression and confusion. However to ask what she is doing, talk about it, even help her, allows us a privileged glimpse of her reality and a clearer understanding of her behaviour and needs. Here a resolution approach to her management aids her quality of life, she is engaged in purposeful activity. In her case indiscriminate use of RO would be devastating, it would reduce her quality of life, she would be imprisoned in a reality she could never understand — ours.

We must therefore accept that once a certain level of dementia is reached, and we are sure of its irreversibility, then RO as a memory therapy becomes neither possible nor useful. This is not to say that we should not use

24-hour RO, for instance labelling rooms, using names and so on, but that it must be a highly individual process geared to that particular person's capabilities, designed to reassure, not to achieve retention. Imagine continually reinforcing to an elderly person that their mother is dead when they have no chance of retaining this information. We would be condemning this person to a life of continual bereavement and serial grief reactions. We must assume, as resolution therapy does, that the behaviour and speech of the demented person holds real meaning for him or her, however nonsensical it may appear to us. So, accept the content, but look for the concealed meaning and focus on the feelings. For instance when they are constantly saying "I must get home to mother" we could reply "You must love your mother very much, tell me about her". The concealed meanings include loneliness, possible grief and isolation. The underlying feelings could then be fear, sadness and despair.

To summarise the research, if the goal is quality of life, then we must assess carefully to decide whether resolution or orientation, or a particular blend of both, is pertinent to that individual. Moreover, whichever technique we choose and whatever groupwork we do with our clients, the basic qualities of unconditional positive regard, warmth and acceptance and the use of Rogerian counselling skills like reflective listening, will determine the value and quality of the relationship and empathy we develop. These are the most significant factors in improving quality of life.

Finally, in realising that memory therapy declines in value as the memory span itself reduces we must also acknowledge that any empathy achieved and sense of well-being brought about by resolution will also be temporary.

Resolution, then, should be regarded as an ongoing approach, as a way of being with dementing elderly people throughout their daily lives.

Many excuses are made for not running groups on long-stay wards or specialist units for profoundly demented people. "We haven't got the time", "the staff are too busy", "we don't have any materials", "you won't get any response", "we tried it before". Usually the factors which militate against success are low staff expectations, poor staff morale, lack of support for enthusiastic staff and insensitive management. Working on such a ward or unit caring for profoundly demented people is physically and mentally draining. It is one of the most undervalued, difficult and underfunded areas of all the caring services. Yet groupwork is not impossible given good management and support. Improving the quality of life for this client group, many of whom have little left they can do for themselves, represents one of the greatest challenges in the caring professions.

The therapeutic programme that follows is simple and many other ideas and activities can be tried once they have settled into the groupwork routine.

This programme is for severely demented people who are resident in long-stay settings, which they are never likely to leave and which are therefore their home. In recognition of staffing levels, the 'heavy' workload and the somewhat diminished physical capabilities of the clientele, it is thought that one group per day is sufficient. Any more will be physically quite tiring and will stretch staffing resources. The workload for staff is generally greater in the morning so it is suggested that the daily group takes place in the afternoons. Many elderly people however like to take a nap in the afternoons and this 'siesta' period should be respected.

How long the group should last will obviously vary; if it is going well fine, if not do not drag it out for the sake of it. The activities in this basic programme normally last around anything between a half to one hour. At the very least two members of staff should run the group, with others joining in as much as is practical and possible. The group leader's sole responsibilitiy must be to the group itself, so that if, for example, members need toileting during the group, then other staff should be available to do this, leaving the group leaders free to keep the group going.

The importance of the group is client participation and stimulation. Group leaders should spend as much time as possible in engaging the patients. For example, if you are making a collage, most time should be spent in showing pictures to individuals and discussing them rather than cutting and pasting the collage. The pictures can be cut out before the group and pasted on quickly throughout the group.

At the very least, those who seem to show no response will get a change of scenery, and a sense of having been involved in something. We have no choice here but to give our clients the benefit of the doubt even though they may give us no indication at all that we have achieved anything. This lack of response, the lack of feedback and hence encouragement is what makes this a most demanding task. However, it can be great fun and thoroughly enjoyable. You just have to be flexible and take the rough with the smooth.

The groupwork programme requires very little in the way of materials. A few music tapes of the 'Singalong-a-Max' music hall variety are the most important items. It is useful to write the words down and make a few song sheets so that there is no excuse for staff not to singalong. A large supply of old magazines for cutting up, scissors, paste and paper are all that is needed for the collage. Additionally, a ball, some bean bags and a waste paper bin will do for games. If you can, use indoor games equipment, such as quoits. If you can take people to a different room, this adds to the sense of occasion, of doing something different and makes the group more of an event. The programme then, runs like this:

MONDAY	
Collage	Pick a theme, for instance, seasons, children, countryside. Cut pictures out, show around the group, talking about each one. What is it? Do you like it? At the end you will have a new picture for the wall. Make the collage as large as possible and use large pictures. Have singalong tapes going in the background.

TUESDAY	
Singalong	Using tapes, unless you have got a piano, and handing out word sheets to willing staff, singalong to the old favourites. Simple musical instruments such as tambourines and maracas can be used to tap out the rhythm. Staff involved should participate fully. Non-participating staff will inhibit others.

WEDNESDAY	
Games	With the singalong tapes going in the background spend some time throwing a soft ball around in a circle engaging people vocally whilst doing it. With your bean bags get people to aim for the waste bin in the middle of the circle. A balloon tossed about the group is usually good fun, four balloons even more so.

THURSDAY	
Singalong	As for Tuesday (combined with several pillow guessing games).

FRIDAY	
Collage	As for Monday (combined with painting).

The reasons for the singalong and collage are that staff quickly pick up the ideas and become proficient, materials and ideas are kept to a minimum and they are by far the most enjoyable sessions. As the programme becomes established the team can broaden out and try different ideas such as art and printing. Wheelchair tyre prints should raise a few eyebrows. Other ideas:

◆ Reminiscence   ◆ Sound games

◆ Exercises   ◆ Dancing

◆ Beauty group   ◆ Skittles

◆ Walks   ◆ Smell games

POSTSCRIPT

Following several months of groups we found that morning and afternoon sessions were needed — people did not get tired and more often than not had more energy than the staff who were the ones in need of a 'siesta' in the afternoon. Many more ideas were tried and were successful . . . we underestimated . . . and many more of the ideas elsewhere in this book can be used. The golden rule is that it is not important what you do as long as you are enthusiastic and convey a sense of occasion and make people smile.

Section G

DAILY LIVING: SKILLS & ADVICE

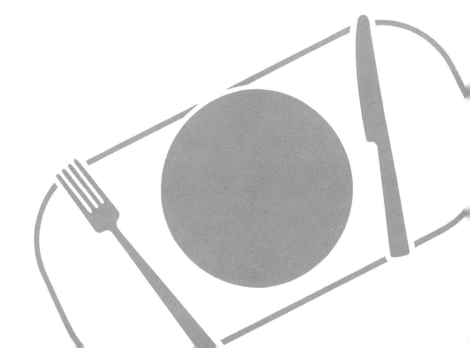

There are several reasons for including cookery and baking in an activity programme:

1 Having a small group prepare a meal gives you the opportunity of assessing and monitoring culinary skills and kitchen safety;

2 Baking sessions in the morning to prepare cakes and biscuits for afternoon tea again gives an opportunity to monitor skills and safety;

3 Perhaps the nicest way of using baking in a groupwork setting is by having a regular social afternoon or tea dance, whereby others are invited and activities planned and cakes, scones and biscuits baked.

An alternative is organising regular jumble or bric-a-brac sales and selling the fruits of your baking — alongside your craftwork. There are plenty of cheap recipe books and a glut of good easy recipes in women's magazines.

Alternatively you can get good information including recipes, from such places as the Flour Advisory Bureau, Milk Marketing Board and Potato Marketing Board.

Another good idea is to list all your members' birthdays and get other members to bake them a cake.

For many people, looking good is synonymous with feeling good. If we think we look a million dollars, or cool, we feel good. We all like being pampered, although men may be more reluctant to admit to it.

Feeling good about the way you look goes a long way to beating the blues and there are many ways in which we can facilitate this. An example will serve to illustrate this.

Having a bath: today I asked one of the staff to give a lady a hand to have a bath. I popped in, "are you decent", to ask if she was OK and she had tears in her eyes saying how she had never been treated so good and how she had never felt she had been cared about so much before. We underestimate the power of a bath. It is not always so cathartic, but it is often a very relaxing experience. A soothing bath, privacy and being pampered never do anyone any harm.

Similarly, having a hair 'do'. The art is to make it into an occasion rather than just throwing a towel around somebody's neck and getting to work with scissors. Isolate a room and get a volunteer hairdresser to set up like a salon. The beams on the clients' faces will tell you how worthwhile it has been.

Manicure and chiropody are frequently overlooked too. Having a manicure is often regarded as a luxury. We should provide it regularly, but keep its status as a luxury. Chiropody is a specialised service that we should lay on — not only is it another opportunity to pamper, it is a profoundly necessary therapy for elderly people.

Make-up sessions are another string to our bow, providing you with another wonderful opportunity to make somebody feel good. Again isolate a special room and make it an event.

Never exclude dementing people from this and similar experiences. A hair wash and perm, followed by a make-up, is not contraindicated by profound memory loss.

A decrease in cognitive ability does not go hand in hand with a decrease in self-respect. It is extremely important that we recognise this fact. The feeling of proudness, of feeling good, the importance of simply having your hair done is far too great to ignore.

I am not of the opinion that washing up tea cups and tidying up are of any great therapeutic value. People have usually let their domestic skills decline for a very good reason. The underlying lack of reasons for living, feelings of worthlessness and declining physical and mental ability are usually explanation enough and enforced practice in domestic competence will only serve to exaggerate feelings of uselessness and frustration if these other areas are not tackled or accepted. If these other factors can be improved then competence in domestic tasks will return to its premorbid level of its own accord. If they cannot be improved then why make our clients suffer undue reinforcement of their incompetence? It is no good just doing it to give people a sense of pride or personal duty; if all you have got to be proud about is being willing and able to pacify your carers by washing up every day then you have got little to be proud about. It is far more important for the carers to concentrate on your ability at just being you. Having said that, there is a role for domestic skills training if those skills will enhance your quality of life and provide you with meaningful satisfaction.

Obviously if you are assessing someone's capabilities then you need to know what they can and cannot do; this can be an important diagnostic tool. Building self-esteem through being a valued group member can also be enhanced through shared tasks. "If we all get stuck in we can have this done in five minutes"; "You wash, I'll dry — OK I'll put them away"; "You sit down, you cooked it." Domestic skills cover huge areas, and, if you move away from the banal washing, tidying and 'how to wear a tie' philosophy, you move into group debates upon different ideas for meals and difficulties with budgeting and shopping, so that alternative strategies and ideas are explored and shared. The group shops, cooks and enjoys its meal. Washing up afterwards is an unavoidable task, probably to be suffered.

All the activities of daily living such as budgeting, getting up in the morning, cooking, shopping, entertaining, finding time to be alone, being safe and so on, can be covered, appraised, improved, better still optimised in social group situations.

Traditional attitudes have a lot to answer for; take, for example, appearance. The high value placed on this by society reflects sadly on our values. If a person's appearance does not bother them and does not leave them open to ridicule and abuse then leave it. There is nothing intrinsically wrong with most forms of dishevelment.

Be aware of why you are encouraging skills development and in whose best interests it is. There can be two aims. First, it can be maintenance of existing skills and restoration of those which are temporarily lost due to feeling downright fed up. Secondly, it may involve learning and practising skills which are not normally part of that individual's sphere of reference. Examples of the latter are: "My husband always looked after the finances"; "My wife always used to do the shopping"; "I picked the horses but my husband always used to go to the bookies."

This more or less speaks for itself and comes under the general heading of health promotion. It forms the basis of a regular session covering a wide range of topics either requested by the clients or deemed useful by the lesser mortals in charge. It aims to make available and disseminate information. More importantly, though, the group chews this information over, exploring the pros and cons, and any alternatives which may arise.

In 1987 the Health Education Council was disbanded and replaced with the Health Education Authority. Each health authority now has a health promotion centre which is a community resource open to all. From these centres you can get leaflets, posters, slide packs, videos, books and much more which all help to back up the message being put across in the group, besides making it more interesting. If need be, the staff at the centre can also help you to run the group as they are experienced at putting across the message.

Below are some ideas for individual sessions. To enhance participation in the groups we use a lot of brainstorming, asking the clients for their opinions on the subject (for instance "What foods are good for you?" and "What foods are bad for you?"). You can also devise small quiz sheets for them to fill in at the beginning of the group then, when you have sifted through the information, go through the quiz. Anyhow here are a few ideas.

DIET AND HEALTHY EATING

You can procure the services of a dietician here; it is always interesting to have a visiting speaker. However there are more than enough props which can be obtained from the health promotion centre to enable you to do it yourself. Basically you are exploring 'what is a healthy diet?' and the importance and sources of its components such as vitamins, minerals, carbohydrates and fats. You can explore the best ways of cooking, look at easy recipes and make some as a group. The organisations listed in the cookery and baking chapter and the leaflets from the health promotion centre all have good recipes, many devised especially with elderly people in mind. At the end of the day people should have a rough idea of what is good for them, what they should avoid and why. The following is a useful small quiz:

1	What percentage of your body weight is water? 30% 50% 70% 90%	**answer** 70%
2	Which of the following has the highest amount of fibre? One Weetabix One slice of wholemeal bread One helping of baked beans One banana	**answer** the beans
3	Which of the following are sugars? maltose glucose fructose dextrose sucrose	**answer** all
4	Rank the following in order of highest to lowest fat: One yogurt One portion of chips Two large sausages One pork pie (small) One small bar of chocolate A small bag of peanuts	6 3 2 1 4 5

ACTIVITIES

5 A glass of coke contains about how many teaspoons of sugar? 1 2 3 4 5	**answer** 4
6 Guinness is good for you True or false	**answer** it depends how much you drink!

EXERCISE

You can use the exercises outlined in chapter 17 here, but it is a good idea to get a physiotherapist to visit to explain the theory behind the exercises, identify a few muscles and advise on what not to attempt. Physiotherapists can also give good advice about the proper methods of lifting. The opportunity also arises for a question and answer session.

TEETH

The services of a dentist or dental hygienist can be procured here and basically what we are about is how to look after our teeth and our dentures. What foods are good for teeth? Why fluoride? What kind of brush? The dentist can explain the different techniques they use and what they can and cannot do. They can also explain the uses of that formidable arsenal of weapons they use. Common complaints and conditions can be explained, such as gingivitis, why our treatment costs so much and how, if at all, we can reduce the costs.

CARE AND MANICURE

You can invite hairdressers, manicurists and beauty therapists to give a talk, and this usually goes down well if it includes demonstrations.

THE BENEFITS MAZE

This is always a useful group. People are never really sure about their pension rights and other benefits to which they may be entitled. The benefits maze is booby trapped with pitfalls, clauses, paragraph 'c's, sub-sections, small print and unintelligible sentences. Ask a welfare worker from your local Citizens Advice Bureau (CAB) to come and give a talk about the work of the CAB and the common problems that arise with pensions and other benefits. You will need plenty of time for the question and answer session afterwards. The best guide you can have for sorting out this maze yourself (the group is bound to raise individual doubts) is an up-to-date copy of the *Disability Rights Handbook*.

SAFETY IN THE HOME

This is a group you can run yourself with some props from the health promotion centre. You can brainstorm all the possible hazards your group can think of, adding your own thoughts or watch a video on the subject to add to your list. Then go through each hazard discussing how they can be avoided.

An extra session could be a talk with a community occupational therapist about aids which can facilitate easier living and adaptations that can be made to the home.

FEET

Obviously you will need a chiropodist, who never fails to gain rapt attention and several referrals. This session covers general care of the feet, what to look for when buying shoes, how to cut your toe nails properly and a discussion of common complaints — corns, bunions, verrucas and their treatment.

THE POLICE AND SECURITY AT HOME

Your local crime prevention officer is your contact here. He or she will inform the group of what measures to take to make their homes secure and thus avoid burglaries. There is also much more advice to be gained, such as how to deal with door-to-door callers who may be bogus. More important, however, is the message that the police do not mind being called, whatever the reason; far better that they attend ten false alarms than people worry and may be at risk. Another useful session is to ask your local beat police officer to come and talk about work; 'A day in the life of . . .' They can highlight the particular difficulties of their patch and its local peculiarities and it is an opportunity for people to get to recognize their local beat officer.

EARS

This is really a group for those with hearing aids. Get an audiologist or technician to come and explain how hearing aids work, what the settings are and how to clean them. Hearing members of the group can also learn in what ways they can adapt their communication in order to aid the hard of hearing. Those whose hearing is ailing can tell the hearers what helps them and what difficulties loss of hearing brings with it so that we have more understanding of their plight. As with any group where you have hearing aid wearers use a 'loop' system if you can. Many hearing aids have a 't' setting. This picks up magnetic waves from a 'loop' of wire connected to a special piece of electrical equipment and a microphone. You can spread the loop around the group and place the microphone in the middle of the group. In this way it amplifies the sound without picking up unwanted noise. It can also be placed near a television or music speaker.

FIRE

Don't panic. A useful beginning to this session is a brainstorm of all the possible fire hazards in the home. The list is phenomenal: chip pans, smoking, worn flexes, hairspray, adaptors, candles, power cuts. Your local fire brigade will put you in touch with a fire prevention officer who can give a thorough breakdown of all the hazards and how they can best be avoided. They can also tell you what to do in the event of fire, and more importantly what not to do, such as not to pour water on a blazing chip pan.

KEEPING WARM

Hypothermia is a killer in our client group, so this is obviously a crucial session. Benefits, meals, clothing, living in one room, all these have to be explored. Reinforce all the strategies for keeping warm. There are many leaflets available. Often, however, at the end of the day it is a question of wearing more clothes, drinking soup and possibly heating one room even if it means moving your bed downstairs. Having said this, help is available of which many people may not be aware. Extra money is available from the Department of Social Security (DSS) in the UK and a social worker will be able to elaborate on this. There are grants for home insulation and several different ways in which you can pay for your fuel; savings stamps and monthly budget payment schemes, for example, help you to spread the cost so that you are not faced with particularly high bills following the winter period when you use more. The type of heating appliances you are using might be particularly costly to run; fan heaters and electric bar fires are examples. The local gas and electricity boards can advise and help with converting to lower cost heating systems and should be able to inform you of any financial help available towards this.

ET AL

There are obviously many other areas to cover; ask your clients for suggestions. A few obvious ones are talks from general practitioners (GPs), social workers, health visitors, community psychiatric nurses, district nurses, vicars, politicians and consumer protection organisations. The focus does not have to be on welfare. Looking after ourselves also involves getting sufficient stimulation and enjoyment from life. Visiting speakers from all walks of life can be invited to address the group. The library will provide you with a list of local clubs and societies which is an invaluable source of useful speakers and, it is hoped, demonstrations. The local photographic society, for example, might come along and put up an exhibition, the local choral society could give a recital. Check what your clients would like to hear about, and what your clients might like to tell the rest of your group about! Local schools and colleges are also a source of talks and demonstrations. Art, music, and cookery students, for example, can all supply knowledge and enthusiasm which is well worth tapping.

This is obviously an important area, it could save your own or someone else's life. Accidents will happen and as you get older they usually happen more frequently. It is a fact that more people die from accidents in the home than from road traffic accidents.

By far the best book to refer to here is the St John's, St Andrew's and Red Cross *First Aid Manual* (see Bibliography). Where possible organise a qualified first aider, from the Red Cross, St John's or your local hospital to help you organise and run these seminars. If you cannot get one, then use the manual. Choose one small area each week, such as burns, cuts, breaks, collapses, head injury, poisoning. Our usual format here is first to go around the group asking members to relate personal experiences of that week's topic. Discuss how it happened and what action was taken. Following this, use the manual to go through the correct procedure for each type of occurrence, for example the different types of burns, different severities of cuts. Whenever possible use props. Get your group to make slings and dress arms severely lacerated by a red felt pen. Finally, to see if it has all sunk in, describe a scenario and get the group to brainstorm what the first aid would be. Make an effort to place the incident in a plausible setting such as a cut in the kitchen, child falling off a bike, someone collapsing in the supermarket, or someone falling down the stairs. The idea is to get them to think about what is available; for example, where there is no first-aid kit, what is a good substitute for a sterile dressing?

Each week as you go through different accidents certain common knowledge will become reinforced, such as ensuring safety from further injuries, eliminating the cause, calling for assistance, dealing with sightseers, being aware of shock, covering distressing sights, getting help and most importantly reassuring the sufferer. A useful adjunct to this group is to have a weekly 'spontaneous' role play. Inform your group that you will be doing this, and then the next week, for instance halfway through the baking session, tell them that you have just knocked a pan of boiling hot soup all down your arm. Carry on role playing until you are satisfied they have mastered the situation. This can be the starting focus of the next week's group. It is all very well talking about it but it is a different kettle of fish when it actually happens.

This is usually a very stimulating group and one in which you can dispel myths. Try and make it topical as well, for example by dealing with hypothermia in winter and sunburn, bites and stings in summer.

By way of example, two useful sessions of mine that were well received and stimulated much discussion were dogs and falls. The coverage of pitbull terrier incidents in the papers stimulated a group on dog bites which included 'What should you do if attacked by a dog?' 'How can you best defend yourself?'

The other session explored a survival issue. 'What do you do if you have a fall, cannot move and cannot get help?'

Section H

PARTIES, PETS & GETTING OUT

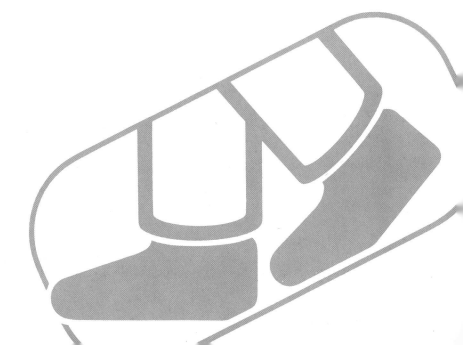

PARTIES AND TRIPS 34

For most of us the year is punctuated with special events and the same should apply in institutional settings. Such events (like holidays and anniversaries) serve not only to locate us within the passing of time, the seasons and our lives but also are the stuff of which memories are made.

Any excuse for a party is a good excuse, seasonal events such as Christmas and Easter, Chinese new year, birthdays, anniversaries and so on are usual, but if you are stuck use Simon Mayo's book *On This Day* and you have an excuse for a party on every day of the year. This, of course, being the anniversary of the invention of the paperclip, gives us another excuse for more, offshoot group-work. Parties, like trips, offer an arena for the practice of social skills; for instance in planning, fundraising, cake making. At parties you will need games to complement your music and food, and you can employ the usual party games, such as musical chairs, if they are appropriate. However, it is often better to focus on less childish pursuits and good quizzes can be devised which are much fun. Two teams doing a noughts and crosses quiz using the full range of your quiz material is great fun, from straightforward questions to smells, noises, pillow guess, what is it, name that tune. A quiz, battle of the sexes, often gives rise to much amusement.

And now for something completely different . . . a good children's 'awful' joke book can get the party off to a groan. Not just for parties though . . . a few really chronic jokes to make people cringe can be used at any group session. After this the group can only get better.

Trips and outings always seem to involve far too much organising, but always turn out to be well worth it. They are also an excuse for subsidiary groupwork, such as shopping for picnic food, making sandwiches, and a 'deciding where to go' group. Wherever you decide upon do not forget the camera and get the group to share the responsibility for navigating. More specifically, museums are obviously good for RO and reminiscence purposes. Traditional farms are also well worth visiting. Wherever you choose to go you are giving your clients fun, experience and an opportunity to practise social skills in a realistic setting, such as cafés. Do not feel that going on a trip has got to be a major event, there is much to be gained from going around your local shopping centre or a large supermarket. The prices will open a few eyes.

Christmas is a great social event and it can act as a focus for groupwork well in advance of its arrival. There are many preparations to be made. You can have a decorations squad working away for a month or two beforehand, a planning team devising and organising parties, and so on. The art and craft section should give you a few ideas — we usually silkscreen our own Christmas cards, make doily snowflakes and design stained glass windows using coloured tissue paper. Large advent calendars can be made from last year's Christmas cards by sandwiching them between two large sheets of card and cutting the doors in the appropriate places. You can make one for yourselves and a few for other people. You can have parties, religious services (do not forget Hanneka), carol singing, games planning, catering — the whole works. There is no real need to go into any more detail here, get your friends and colleagues to shine by dreaming up decoration ideas like putting glitter on pine cones. I usually buy every woman's magazine under the sun just before Christmas, because they are full of useful ideas. What I can do now, though, is give you a Christmas quiz to add a seasonal flavour to your Christmas party. But let us not forget the Christmas tipple — start a home brew group in early January so that by Christmas you have mastered the art of producing something faintly palatable!

THE CHRISTMAS QUIZ

1 Good King Wenceslas was King of which country?
Bohemia — now Czechoslovakia

2 What was a yule log?
A large log, lit on Christmas eve and which continued to burn throughout the Christmas period

3 What gifts did the three Wise Men bring?
Gold, frankincense and myrrh

4 What is myrrh?
Used in the East for incense and embalming

5 On the 12 days of Christmas my true love sent to me:
    (i)   A partridge in a pear tree
    (ii) Two turtle doves
    (iii) Three french hens
    (iv) Four calling birds
    (v)   Five gold rings
    (vi) Six geese a laying
    (vii) Seven swans a swimming
    (viii) Eight maids a milking
    (ix) Nine ladies dancing
    (x)   Ten lords a leaping
    (xi) Eleven pipers piping
    (xii) Twelve drummers drumming.

6 The annual Trafalgar Square Christmas tree is donated by which country?
Norway

7 Who was the King of Judea when Jesus was born?
Herod

8 Here we come a wassailing; what is a wassail?
From the Saxon 'wass hael', meaning 'good health'.
Now though it means carol singing for most people

9 Boxing Day is the feast of which saint?
Saint Stephen

10 From which carols do the following lines come?

(a)	The cattle are lowing	Away in a Manger
(b)	Sing choirs of angels, sing in exaltation	O Come all ye Faithful
(c)	In fields where they lay	The First Noel
(d)	Deep and crisp and even	Good King Wenceslas
(e)	All is calm, all is bright	Silent Night
(f)	All seated on the ground	While Shepherds Watched
(g)	In a manger for his bed	Once in Royal David's City
(h)	Let nothing you dismay	God Rest ye Merry Gentlemen
(i)	Peace on earth and mercy mild	Hark, the Herald Angels Sing
(j)	The rising of the sun and the running of the deer	The Holly and the Ivy

11 Who wrote *A Christmas Carol?*
Charles Dickens

12 Which astrological sign does Christmas day fall on?
Capricorn — from 22 December to 19 January

13 On 25 December 1777 Captain Cook discovered a small island in the Pacific. What did he call it?
Christmas Island (There is another in the Indian Ocean discovered in 1643.)

14 Who sang *White Christmas?*
Bing Crosby

15 Born on Christmas Eve 1899 he starred in *The Maltese Falcon* and *Casablanca.*
Humphrey Bogart

16 Born on Boxing Day 1883 he was the leader of the Chinese Communist Party.
Mao Tse Tung

17 In Dickens's *A Christmas Carol* who was a miserly man who saw the ghost of Christmas past?
Ebenezer Scrooge

18 Spell Wenceslas

19 Who wrote the traditional Christmas music called *The Messiah?*
Handel

20 New Year's Eve in Scotland is called —
Hogmanay

21 The custom of decorating Christmas trees was introduced to this country by —
Prince Albert (He brought it from Germany when he married Queen Victoria)

22 What are the names of the three Wise Men?
Melchior, Balthazar and Caspar

23 From which country does kissing under the mistletoe originate?
England — seventeenth century

24 If a child posts a letter to Father Christmas, c/o The North Pole, will he get a reply?
Yes — a team in Edinburgh replies to all such letters and signs them Father Christmas

25 Who is the original Father Christmas?
St Nicholas — fourth century; famous for his love of
children and generosity

26 Where do turkeys come from in the wild?
Mexico

27 Why is Boxing Day so called?
Because employers used to give money in 'boxes' on
St Stephen's Day. Hence Christmas boxes

28 What tree is traditionally 'the' Christmas tree?
Norway spruce (*picea abies*)

29 Why do we find robins on Christmas cards?
Because they have a red breast and postmen used to wear
red jackets

30 You are driving a bus, at the first stop three men and a girl
with a dog get on, at the second stop one man gets off and
two men get on, at the third stop the girl with the dog gets
off and two ladies get on, at the fourth stop only one man
gets off . . . how old is the driver?
You should know — you are the driver!

If you are lucky enough to have some outdoor gardening space then a small group could be set up with a view to tending it regularly. You could grow your own vegetables or just plant a few flowers, bulbs or whatever just for something to look at. Then come the spring and summer you will have somewhere nice to sit and have your groups and tea.

You should be able to recruit a local gardener to give you guidance and who can come in for a few hours a week.

Try to derive added benefit by making your garden into one that will attract wildlife. Try planting natural wild flowers and plants which will encourage insects. Buddleia bushes, for instance, attract tortoise-shell butterflies.

A bird table and bird bath will also add greatly to your enjoyment of the garden. Get a few good bird posters and keep a yearly list of birds seen in your patch.

Having no outdoor area does not mean you have to miss out. You can have window boxes either inside or outside. Planting bulbs such as daffodils outside in a container and hyacinths indoors can be very rewarding. A good book on house plants should provide a mountain of ideas.

Tomatoes are a personal favourite growing on a sunlit window sill; gradually watching them ripen gives a sense of achievement.

Even better though is growing your own oak trees. In the late autumn when the acorns begin to drop go for a walk in the woods and collect half a dozen acorns in which the first root has just broken through. Carefully place these on 3 cm (1 inch) of soil in a tray or other container and cover lightly with a little more soil. Place in a dark warm place (I used the airing cupboard) and keep them moist. By spring they should be small saplings 20 cm (9 inches) or more high. Transplant them into larger pots as they get taller.

Other ideas for green-fingered clients are the small kits you can buy for indoor gardens. They are aimed at children but some of them are very good.

Introducing pets into an environment of elderly people will be one of the best things you ever do. Pets offer companionship and acceptance, they have no regard for our taboos and social restrictions. They also stimulate the sense of touch. The enjoyment pets can give greatly helps in improving the quality of life for clients in both day care and residential settings.

A certain amount of common sense is needed, however, as some people do not like animals and some have acute phobias. Dogs with a high energy level should be avoided for obvious reasons.

If you cannot keep a pet in your particular context then organise regular visits from dog owners. Other pets can be used, but there is something about dogs that seems to bring out the best in us. I think it is the eyes and their total acceptance of any of us. These regular visits give people a pleasurable experience. They can draw out isolated individuals and increase their responsiveness. It provides the opportunity for us to reminisce about our own pets and experiences with animals. The antics of the dogs and just the sheer joy of patting them can animate and lift our mood. They are a catalyst for social behaviour, getting people talking and sharing their joy. Withdrawn and confused people can become alert and communicative. They smile more, talk more and generally become more alert. Indeed it has been said that . . .

"Dogs and cats can be made available for more hours at a much lower cost and in greater numbers than psychiatrists and nurses."

Section I

CONSIDERATIONS

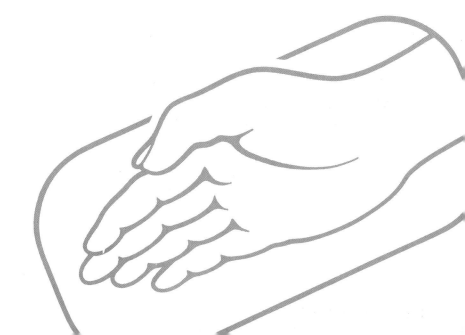

38

Ifs, buts, maybes, howevers, althoughs and other sundry problems usually occur in groupwork! That is to say that if the above do not occur, then you are doing it wrong. The problems that can occur with groupwork are a desperately difficult thing to write about, our client group throws more spanners in the works than one would normally have to deal with. But let us not mystify the whole thing by saying you need to have done such and such a course, or need to have undergone x years of training. There is an awful lot of professional mystery flying about at the moment which, to protect various people's status, will tell you otherwise. There is no training like supervised practice, which means you will not learn much in a classroom, the only way to learn is by getting your face covered in large quantities of egg and your feet very wet. There are no rules, only guidelines that can be passed on from those who have washed their faces.

If you get a group of elderly confused people together and have a laugh, enjoy yourselves and come out smiling you have done good groupwork. Place that scenario on the monotony of a long-stay psychogeriatric ward and you can realize the importance of it. An active groupwork programme can break up the day and provide identifiable times at which 'something will happen'. Groups can teach us a lot about elderly people . . . that they are stimulating, intelligent and individual. So the first rule of groupwork is to respect your group.

It is important and advisable that you do not undertake groupwork on your own; no-one is that skilled. You will miss an awful lot of what is going on and what interactions take place because you will be too busy keeping the group going and focused in the way you wish it. Co-workers can see more clearly who was left out, who dominated, who fell asleep, who was overawed and who felt insecure. They are also invaluable in supporting you during the group, helping you to maintain the flow and aiding the quiet, withdrawn and those with sensory deficiencies. We can learn a lot about our clients in groups but we cannot pick up on everything if we are alone.

Apart from not being on your own you need to know what you are doing. So do not call groups social skills groups when they are for instance merely a 'practising washing up group'. You need to be clear in your aims, so that you can refocus the group if this is not happening. If assistance is not available you must limit the group's numbers. You also need to be familiar with your topic and prepare yourself. The group is not the place to try something out for the first time. Use your fellow workers. More plainly if you are running a current affairs group do not spend half the session flicking through the paper looking for something interesting. Spend ten minutes previously marking headlines, pictures and so on.

Keeping the group focused is not as easy as it sounds. Digression has a knack of steering you off track without you seeing it. Digression however is not always a bad thing. Total non–participation, complete silence, the occasional grunt, you being the only one left awake, you falling asleep, these are all far worse. Peaceful, but far worse. If a group wants to digress and that is where they want to go, fine. But if it is a ploy to avoid an issue then you must point this out to the group and confront them. If you do not point it out and you allow the group to waffle on, what do they learn? If you confront it, then they at least recognize their avoidance and you have refocused onto the issue. Why have we avoided it? What can't we face? What shall we do about it?

Another problem arises when clients do not use the 'group' but address all their comments to you. You are a facilitator, an enabler, not a leader, not the chairperson, not the judge or teacher. Explain this to the group and point out that questions should be addressed to the group as a whole. You are not there to provide answers but to try and help the group come up with their own. Beware also group leaders and co-workers talking too much; if the leader dominates the group, it is wasted. This can be a problem if you are using volunteers and staff who are unfamiliar with group-work and your aims. It is partly your fault for not vetting your co-workers sufficiently or not giving them sufficient insight beforehand. However, as I said they have to learn, and it is best if they can relate their mistakes to a real group experience and turn it into a valuable learning experience. Intervene subtly, give control back to the group and go through the experience afterwards with the person concerned.

Non participation comes in many guises and has many root causes. Boredom, irrelevance, shyness, fear of confronting awkward issues, fear of being wrong, fear of being rejected. It can show itself via silence, one word answers, digression, misplaced joviality, sabotage, walking out, tears, and a host of other ways. Non participation should never be ignored, it often means that there is a serious issue crying out for confrontation. Your skill as a facilitator lies in confronting the non participation without putting any individual on the spot. "I have a feeling that the group is avoiding something here, maybe we should think about this and explore it a little." Silences should be allowed to go on, they give time for quiet reflection and raise the awareness of the group members that "Yes, this is indeed a touchy and important area". Breaking 'awkward' silences will only feed back to the group that you too feel scared about this issue and do not know how to deal with it and will make the group feel unsafe. If you cannot handle it how can they? You should make the group feel safe, that you recognize the importance that this silence places on the issues at hand and feed this back to the group; this will boost the confidence of the group and help the issue to be explored.

It is important to be aware also that silences often reflect the lack of group cohesion. You may have asked the group to confront awkward issues too early. It may be that you feel this too and are unwittingly showing uneasiness, in which case the group may be protecting you! Misplaced joviality and deliberate sabotage, "This is stupid, let's go", should be confronted in a similar manner. Explore the reasons behind it and confirm the difficulties the issue raises, offer your view of the reason for the sabotage and ask the group to confront your view.

If members walk out of the group you must accept that, OK they may feel very unsafe with the issues the group is handling, but also walking out of a group is not an easy thing to do either. Ask the group what they want to do about it. If they don't want to do anything you must explore this further, it too may be sabotage, but if they do, then ask one of them (if no-one volunteers) to go and ask the member to return saying that they are a valued member and are missed and the group is concerned about them . . . but only if it is true. If it is not then further exploration is necessary. The groups we are envisaging here will seldom, if ever, get this 'heavy' but never underestimate the volume of feeling you can create. It is advisable to be aware at all times what a powerful instrument a group can be.

Clients arguing can be dealt with in similar ways. It could be sabotage, but if it is not it has raised issues which need exploring — so ensure they are explored. Often one or several clients will dominate the group and you have a duty to try to point out to the group that this is occurring; if this is not pointed out it is a green light to that member that it is OK. Similarly, eight conversations going on at once shows little respect for the group and its supposed focus. Confront this and control it bearing in mind that sabotage may not be deliberate. This is where withdrawn members get steam rollered and you must make a conscious effort to get the group (not you) to allow them time and space. Everyone should be given the opportunity to speak. The quiet and withdrawn should be given praise and feedback that their contribution, however small, is valued.

Never hurry a group; do not get upset if results are slow in coming. The rules of good counselling apply. Be impartial, do not opinionate or judge, use open-ended questions not those which demand only one word answers. Do not expect too much of groups too soon. The 'rules' of groups are not easy to become familiar with and it will take a while, for example, for the group to stop putting their questions directly to you.

Anger is a feeling which is often experienced in groups and you must try and appreciate whether it is realistic and pertinent to the group or relates to 'outside' non-group issues. If it is realistic, you must stick with it and explore it. If not, then you need to point this out. It is a useful sabotage tool so draw the group in and say what effect it is having on the group. If the group is dogged by a consistent disrupter then remember that group membership is voluntary. That member is free to leave the group, but should they wish to stay they must respect the group's rules and aims and that they have a duty to the other members of the group not to dominate and sabotage.

You too should respect the group and recognise the privilege you hold as their facilitator. You should be fit to run the group. They are not easy and if you are tired this will damage the group's cohesion and your own credibility. It is important also to set time limits and adhere to them. Start on time, some members may have geared themselves up to speak in the group — a half hour's delay could destroy their nerve and they will hold you responsible. Finish on time so that if difficult issues are raised the group knows exactly when the pressure will be off.

With special regard to groups with confused clients or those suffering various degrees of dementia it is important that you fully evaluate each individual beforehand. We all have different abilities and skill levels. The activity and topic must fit these levels, so do not have too wide a variation of cognitive ability in these groups otherwise, as we have said before, half will be frustrated and the other half will be insulted. Many dementia sufferers, especially in the early years, retain a degree of insight and recognize that they have deficiencies. In a group situation they may fear that these will become obvious and will be exposed and this can lead, obviously, to reluctance to join in. To understand this is crucial.

Research has shown that concentration has a tendency to fall following lunch. Concentration declines for as much as two hours. Be aware of this and run any remotely intense groups early on in the day. The period after lunch, especially for our clients, should be regarded as a siesta and should be used to refocus our attention on our major goal — that being alive should be fun.

We must also add a word of caution about groupworkers and volunteers. Using volunteers is good, we all have something to give, but beware the volunteer taking over and going on about their holiday or family life, thereby depressing the rest of the group. Volunteers need reminding in whose interests the group exists. Beyond this — beware professionals. You can train in groupwork, but no amount of training will make you a good groupworker if you are not receptive to change and experience. We are all still learning. You are either that kind of person or you are not. Nothing in the world can make an extrovert a good listener.

ONE TO ONE

Finally, we must not become over dependent on groups. It is all too easy when engrossed in group living or day care situations to forget about the value of one to one, face to face, good, honest, private talking.

Not everyone can respond to or feel comfortable in a group situation. It is important to recognize this, respect and cater for it. Even those who seemingly thrive on groups and appear to draw much benefit and strength from them need space to breathe and time to reflect. There should always be the opportunity to spend time in building one-to-one relationships. Some people will never respond in groups, we are not all comfortable in company, nor should we be expected to be so. There are some things which can only be shared within the context of a special relationship and we must never lose sight of this. The group is not the answer to all our problems.

One of the most important things you are ever likely to do if you are working with elderly mentally ill and infirm people is to set up a carers' support group. They are the advocates and the voice of the sufferer. They are also the advocates and the voice of their own plight. Support groups can fulfil a multitude of needs ranging from being information exchanges to just somewhere you can vent your frustration. The giving and taking of mutual support by people in the same situation provides the opportunity for expression of carers' feelings of frustration, anger, resentment and guilt. All too often people cope in isolation leaving themselves open to becoming ill themselves with depression and exhaustion.

But the groups can also be a source of practical support and information and an ideas exchange. Speakers can be arranged to pass on specialist knowledge, management of difficult behaviours, medicines, benefits and so on. The existence of the group itself will reduce feelings of isolation and shared discussion will promote familiarity with local services. Strategies for dealing with common problems and behaviours can be brainstormed and supplemented with professional know-how. The roles of various different agencies and services, such as GPs, social workers, community psychiatric nurses, MIND, Age Concern, psychiatrists, can all be explored and clarified.

The most important factor though is purely mutual support. Chats over cups of tea after the discussion or speaker are often the most beneficial parts of the meeting for carers. "My wife's just like that", "I know, don't tell me, it's terrible"!

Such groups have benefits for care workers too. They obviously give an insight into the manifold problems and worries of carers. Our services should in part be based on their needs, how better to find out about them! The groups can also act as an early warning system for signs of carers under strain and in need of imminent relief. A worker skilled in this field can be of benefit by seeing early on and intercepting those who may be feeling guilty at not coping as adequately as everyone else seems to be doing. It would be easy for a quiet person to attend the meeting, listen and go home feeling drastically incompetent and thoroughly depressed because everyone else is doing so magnificently. Seek out the meek.

Meetings are always difficult to arrange to suit everyone's convenience. Many of the carers themselves are elderly, do not drive and cannot get anyone to look after their loved one whilst they attend. You have got far more resources than they have so try and explore lunch times or afternoon meetings so nobody has to come out in the dark and try to provide transport yourself. Also either help to arrange sitters or organize a sufferers' group and staff for it to coincide with the carers' group.

Finally, let us just explore a few of the states of mind a carer can be faced with:

Confusion: when a loved one's personality starts to disintegrate, the previously alert and loving partner becomes a dull but short-tempered, irritable and aggressive person and you have no idea they are dementing or what dementia is.

Disgust: and horror at incontinence and failing social skills, the decline of dignity and apparent self-respect of a previously fastidious partner.

Anger: Dementia is a living hell. Let us not get sentimental. Your lover is unrecognizable. This is not the person you married. You are suffering a bereavement nobody will acknowledge, you cannot express your grief. Why US? Why ME? All the things you had planned to do together in your retirement, all you had worked and saved for is blown away on something intangible that cannot be shared. Anger at the lack of recognition, the lack of help from social services, the National Health Service (NHS), family and a GP who all too often says there is nothing that can be done.

Strain: on your job, on your family. The fear of social disgrace, of being socially ostracised. What will the neighbours say? What will the grandchildren think?

Loss: of friends, of lover, partner, holidays, money, hobbies, time, status, support, conversation, sex, shared laughter, shared anything, strength, appetite, willpower, sleep, time to yourself, time to reflect, loss of future.

Fear: will it happen to me, the children, the grandchildren? What will people think, what will they say, can I cope, will I give up, what will I do, who will understand, how will I manage, will I have to sell the house, who will stay my friend?

Guilt: I can't cope, I don't understand, I'm useless, I don't know, I can't love you . . .

"Talking about my generation . . ."

I was a teenage 'Who' freak, but I am alright now! One of the questions constantly, no, intermittently occurring to me is that if I suffer memory loss and if I ever find myself in a reminiscence group, then will the people running the group be in tune with what was important to me. If they highlight the seventies will I be subject to the torture of constant reference and tapes of Boney M, the Sweet, Gary Glitter and the like. It is a nightmare that my individual tastes and preferences will be ignored and that I will be expected to get excited about listening to pathetic, run of the mill, middle of the road (chirpy chirpy cheep cheep — remember that?) songs that the organizers enthuse about as being representative of that era. I hope this underlies what we have been saying about getting a good history from family and friends and getting to know what made your client tick. What made each an individual? Some of the old, 'we'll meet again', 'pack up your troubles' type songs make some of your clients sick, they were anti-war in politics and jazz oriented in music. Know thy client and their individuality.

Know your people as individuals, not just as age groups or locals, do not automatically band them together.

One thing we have found recently is that our reminiscence materials relating to the twenties are getting out of date. It is 1993 and at the end of the twenties our client group was aged roughly 15 and they cannot remember the twenties very much at all. Our props therefore need radically updating. We are fortunate over the last 20 years, and even more so now, to have been blessed with a plethora of glossy magazines. These are the RO and reminiscence material of the future. (Is anybody cutting out pictures and making scrap books in preparation?)

We ought to be making our own reminiscence books, because only we know what we are interested in, we are in the best position to judge our generation's concerns. Life is easier though for future groupworkers; you can now buy videos of every year and find good photographic books on every year so perhaps we will benefit in our later years from today's communications technology.

They have just opened a rock and roll museum, waxworks and hall of fame in Picadilly Circus, London. This is a reminiscence tool par excellence of the future. Like a good insurance salesman I am saving now for the future.

This is the most important chapter in the book — where to get help. The best and most obvious sources are your friends and fellow workers. . . many hands make light work . . . two heads are better than one. It is heartening to find out what other people know.

Other useful sources are:

Health Advisory Service
Known locally as health promotion centres. These can give you leaflets, posters, videos, slides, books and so on, and provide you with speakers for a health promotion group — dieticians, chiropodists for instance.

Citizens Advice Bureau
Provides up-to-date benefits leaflets and speakers who know the ins and outs of the pensions and benefits maze.

Antiques and Book Fairs
This is a most useful and under used resource in our field of work. It is also a very pleasant way of spending some time and money. The quantity and quality of RO and reminiscence material you can pick up here is over-whelming. Old postcards are one of the few surviving sources of what places used to look like and usually what is written on the back is interesting too. I have got many that were obviously written by young men destined for war service and they provide volumes of feeling in a few short lines. Old cigarette cards are good as well. At antique fairs you can pick up cheap knick-knacks that stimulate recall for a particular era. One of the best and still cheapest materials are old film 'year books' that have large glossy pictures of stars from the forties and fifties onwards. Old sports books are still cheap as well.

Tourist Information
Along with travel agents this is your cheapest (free) source of good, large colour pictures. State your purpose and you will usually be well catered for.

Museums
Obviously a place to visit but also a source of artefacts and local history information. You may be able to borrow unusual objects, old books and postcards and so on.

Newspapers
Many local newspapers do a series on yesteryear which is worth organising into a scrapbook. If you write to them you may be able to get better quality pictures than those published.

Schools and Colleges
These are a source of hidden talent, from using primary school children's paintings to having sixth form art students taking sessions with you. Further education colleges can also be useful; for instance drama and music students can run workshops.

Clubs and Societies
These are legion and you can almost guarantee that whatever the interest there is a local society for it. Photographic societies can be asked to produce a 'local landmarks' series, besides giving talks and exhibitions. Other useful categories include poets, collectors, animal groups, and music.

Libraries
Besides books and records for borrowing your local library will also often sell old books and music at ridiculous prices. But above all your library, more especially your librarian, will be a source of much important information on sources,

resources, and contacts, and what they do not know they can usually find out. They will have a list of local clubs, societies and voluntary organisations.

Art Galleries
Again obviously for visits but also for old postcards and posters.

Photocopiers
One of the most useful pieces of equipment you will ever come across. Their ability to enlarge things like small print, maps, small photos and designs make them a godsend.

Old Magazines
Get as many people as possible to collect them for you or organize raids on local paper recycling skips, remembering to recycle those with which you have finished. These are visual aids covering art, wildlife, places, famous people, lifestyle, nostalgia and providing collage material.

USEFUL CONTACTS

Age Concern
Astral House, 1268 London Road, London SW16 4ER

Alzheimer's Disease Education & Referral Center, PO Box 8250, Silver Spring, Maryland 20907–8250, USA

Alzheimer's Disease Society
2nd Floor, Gordon House, 10 Greencoat Place, London SW1P 1PH

Carers National Association
20–25 Glasshouse Yard, London EC1A 4JN

Centre for Policy on Ageing
25-31 Ironmonger Row, London EC1V 3QP

National Dairy Council
5–7 John Princess Street, London W1M 0AP

Disabled Living Foundation
380-384 Harrow Road, London W9 2HW

Flour Advisory Bureau
21 Arlington Street, London N14 5BD

Help the Aged
16–18 St James's Walk, London EC1R 0BE

MIND
Granta House, 15–19 Broadway, Stratford, London E15 4BQ

Nottingham Rehab (equipment)
Ludlow Hill Road, West Bridgford, Nottingham NG2 6HD

Potato Marketing Board
Broadfield House, 4 Between Towns Road, Cowley, Oxon OX4 3NA

S & S Worldwide
75 Mill Street, PO Box 513, Colchester, Connecticut 06415, USA

Ulsvercroft Large Print Books Limited (list of titles available on request)
The Green, Bradgate Road, Anstey, Leicester LE7 7FU

University of the Third Age National Office
26 Harrison Street, London WC1H 8JG

Winslow Press Limited (Large selection of activity, reminiscence and related materials)
Telford Road, Bicester, Oxon OX6 0TS

Do not forget:

1 Your local health promotion centre

2 Library

3 Telephone book — the London Business edition is especially useful in the UK. If you look under London, British and National in a British telephone directory, for example, you will find the headquarters of almost every major society who may or may not be of any use to you — but for the cost of a few stamps and a well-worded letter you may well be rewarded. Do not just say, 'please can you send me some pictures', but explain why you need them, for instance what RO and reminiscence are all about.

4 The other thing to do of course is to use the major national companies. For whatever subject you need materials or resources find a company that deals in it and send them an explanatory letter. For instance 'travel' suggests British Rail, London Bus and National Bus Company, Raleigh Cycles, Honda, Ford to name but a few.

BIBLIOGRAPHY

Argyle M, *The Psychology of Interpersonal Behaviour*, Penguin Books, London, 1967.

Babins L, 'A Humanistic Approach to Old-Old People: A General Model' in *Activities, Adaptation and Ageing*, pp57-63, Haworth Press, New York, 1986.

Beck A & Greenberg R, *Coping with Depression*, Institute for Rational Living, New York, 1974.

Bender M, Norris A & Bauckham P, *Groupwork with the Elderly — Principles and Practice*, Winslow Press, Bicester, 1987.

Bleathman C & Morton I, 'Validation Therapy with the Demented Elderly', *Journal of Advanced Nursing* 13, pp511-514, 1988

Brandes D & Phillips H, *The Gamesters Handbook*, Vols 1 & 2, Tyneside Growth Centre, 54 St Georges Terrace, Newcastle upon Tyne, 1977.

Briscoe T, *Develop an Activities Programme*, Winslow Press, Bicester, 1991.

Brook P et al, 'Reality Orientation — a Therapy for Psychogeriatric Patients', *British Journal of Psychiatry*, 127, pp42-45, 1975.

Burton M, 'Reality Orientation for the Elderly — A Critique', *Journal of Advanced Nursing*, 7, pp427-433, 1982.

Calverley C, *The Family Quizbook*, Penguin, London, 1980.

Carruthers C, *Personal Care*, Winslow Press, Bicester, 1987.

Evans L et al, *Something to Look Forward to — An Evaluation of a Travelling Day hospital for the Elderly Mentally Ill*, Report No. 15, Social Services Research Unit, Portsmouth, 1986.

Feil N, *Validation — the Feil Method*, Edward Feil Publications, Cleveland, USA, 1982.

First Aid Manual, — *Emergency Procedures for Everyone at Home, at Work or at Leisure*, Dorling Kindersley, London, 1987. (Reprinted frequently. This is the authorised first-aid manual of the St John's Ambulance Society and the Red Cross.)

Foster P (ed) *Therapeutic Activities with the Impaired Elderly*, Haworth Press, New York, 1986.

Fuchs E, 'How Teachers Help Children to Fail', Chapter 3 in Keddie N (ed), *Tinker, Tailer ... the Myth of Cultural Deprivation*, Penguin, London, 1973.

Godlove C, Richard L & Rodwell G, 'Time for Action', *Community Care*, University of Sheffield, Joint Unit for Social Science Research, 1980.

Holden U P & Woods R T, *Reality Orientation — Psychological Approaches to the 'Confused' Elderly*, Churchill Livingstone, Edinburgh, 1982.

Hong C S, *Activities Digest*, Winslow Press, Bicester, 1986.

Leitch M, *World War Two Songs*, Wise Publications, London, undated.

Mayo S, *On This Day in History*, Armada, London, 1989.

Merchant M & Saxby P, 'Reality Orientation — a way forward', *Nursing Times*, Aug 12, pp1442-1445, 1981.

BIBLIOGRAPHY

Page A, *Babies Names*, Elliot-Rightway Books, Kingswood, Surrey, 1973

Papadopoulos A, *Counselling Carers*, Winslow Press, Bicester, 1990.

Robertson J, *Personal Safety*, Winslow Press, Bicester, 1987.

Rodgers C, *Client Centred Therapy*, Houghton Mifflin, New York, 1965.

Sampson A & Sampson S, *The Oxford Book of Ages*, Oxford University Press, 1988.

Sheridan C, *Failure Free Activities for the Alzheimer's Patient*, Cottage Books, San Francisco, 1987.

Sherman M, *The Reminiscence Quiz Book*, Winslow Press, Bicester, 1991.

Stokes G & Goudie F, 'Counselling Confused Elderly People' in Stokes G & Goudie F (eds), *Working with Dementia*, Winslow Press, Bicester, 1990.

The Concise Oxford Dictionary of Quotations, Oxford University Press, 1981.

Woods R T, 'Reality Orientation and Staff Attention', *British Journal of Psychiatry*, 134, pp502-506, 1979.

Zepelin H et al, 'Evaluation of a Year Long Reality Orientation Program', *Journal of Gerontology*, 36, pp70-77, 1981.